Probiotic

vs

Commercial Probiotics

by Becky Plotner

Probiotic Foods vs Commercial Probiotics
by Becky Plotner

ISBN: 9781097440597
Published by The Dancing Rhino LLC

Other titles by Becky Plotner
GAPS, Stage by Stage, With Recipes
Joyous Song, The Proverbs 31 Woman
A Walking Tour of Lincoln Road, South Beach
Ocean Drive Guidebook, Ask a Local
The Fontainebleau, Miami & Las Vegas (Ask a Local)

I wish to thank my loving husband Kevin, and my children Gage and Cooper, who supported my efforts to write this book. I'd also like to thank all the practitioners and clients that have helped me in so many ways. I am grateful to you all.

Contents

Forward

I had a woman come up to me, she had been suffering from irritable bowel for many years. She had done everything short of an operation. She said she started eating sauerkraut and within two weeks it was gone.

Becky has shown me her book on probiotics and gut health and I thought it was just excellent – one of the best I've seen, and believe me a lot of books come across my desk. I just thought it was excellent. I'm particularly pleased on the emphasis on food, using fermented foods. I was very interested in what she had to say about probiotic supplements and some of the additives they contain.

- Sally Fallon, author and President of The Weston A. Price Organization

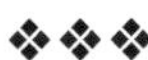

Becky Plotner is an experienced Certified GAPS Practitioner and a person who went through a tremendous journey of healing and recovery from chronic illnesses not only in her family members but also in herself.

She has the kind of life experience which makes the best health practitioner!

In her book Probiotic Foods vs Commercial Probiotics, she has done the hard work of reviewing solid scientific literature on the use of probiotics for different clinical applications. She has compiled information not only about commercial probiotics, but very importantly about homemade fermented foods, such as kefir, yogurt, fermented breast milk and fermented vegetables.

This book will be a valuable tool for clinicians, Certified GAPS Practitioners and other health practitioners to deepen their knowledge about how to use probiotics in clinical settings.

The book is full of useful clinical gems, and I am sure that even a seasoned clinician will find something new to learn in its pages.

I would like to thank Becky for doing this work! I warmly recommend this book!

- Dr. Natasha Campbell-McBride,
MD, MMedSci (neurology), MMedSci (nutrition)
Author of *Gut and Psychology Syndrome*

Introduction

Probiotic foods have traditionally been staples in many countries. Recent studies on probiotics and probiotic foods are showing amazing findings. It was fascinating to see some of the studies on food based probiotics and then compare them to commercial probiotics. When studying each food, different techniques are often used to test what the probiotic food can do inside your body, and what pathogens each one counteracts. Studying commercial probiotics, or using commercial probiotics, is a totally different subject.

Commercial probiotics are supplements. The supplement industry is a self-regulated industry, which means that the manufacturer determines what is good to put in the supplement. After recently writing an article on commercial probiotics that don't rank high, I received a phone call from the president and CEO of a supplement company bearing his name. He told me that the starch they used in the probiotic caused it to maintain a shelf life that made it profitable. He made it very clear that if anything was negatively said about his company or his products, that I would receive a world of hurt and I would be shut down, saying, "You have no idea what I can do to you, to shame you, to discredit you, to burn through your money in court like it was water."

The article was removed.

Finding out how commercial manufacturers make their probiotics is not easy; as each told me, "That's proprietary information." After contacting countless companies, the hope of obtaining information was becoming bleak. Only two companies gave any insight into how they manufactured their probiotics, both of which said the information was not to be published connected to their names.

One company said they grow their probiotics on food scraps and put the by-product into a liquid medium for consumption.

Another company said they grow their probiotics on bits of food, where the probiotic bubbles up on top. The probiotic layer is scraped off, dried on large sheets, powdered, and put into capsules or containers.

When I set out on the adventure of putting this book together, my intention was simple. I wanted to know if home-brewed probiotic foods, like kraut juice, sauerkraut, milk kefir, fermented garlic, fermented fish, fermented beans, beet kvass, kombucha, and others, were just as good as commercial probiotics, which cost hundreds of dollars. We didn't have the extra money to spend, and I was desperate. Honestly, the findings were shocking.

We no longer fear getting sick. We no longer rely on the traditional medical model when someone gets sick; instead, we support our systems properly with fermented foods. When someone feels they are picking up a cold, flu, or other illness, we simply turn to the probiotic food that addresses that ailment, according to the NIH studies listed in *Probiotic Foods vs Commercial Probiotics*. Most recently, my husband suffered from itchy eczema, which grew into a horrific fire that itched and irritated his skin so profusely that it was angry, purple, and he was going mad inside his head with itching. He took four hot showers a day to calm the incessant itch. When he told me about it, I didn't trust the findings and ordered over $350 of commercial probiotics, which he finished in 2 weeks. After it barely soothed his fire, we began addressing the issues with the probiotic food specific to his issue. He drank 2 quarts of it a day, and it was 80 percent soothed the first day and totally gone shortly thereafter.

Probiotics are tools in the toolbox, to be used for different situations. Knowing which ones to use at each given time is a valuable skill everyone needs to know.

- Becky Plotner, ND, tdnl nat, CGP, D.PSc

Probiotics

Nearly everyone is sick today. Food restriction, for most, is not optional; it is imperative. This is not a trend in society; it is illness and digestive disease that has grown to an overwhelming crisis. We are continually seeing foods beginning to hurt, pain escalating for the person, and bodily functions beginning to malfunction.

Food elimination is usually the beginning. A food hurts, and it is removed. The problem with eliminating foods is that the person ends up taking out more, and more, and more food options as the years pass. For most, the eventual outcome is a very limited diet. Some end up with only one or three foods that they can eat.

Removing foods is not the answer. Rebuilding the microbiome is the goal.

A balanced microbiome is acquired by feeding the resident microbes on a regular basis. Feeding happens with real food, in its natural state, with a consistent focus on continual introduction of probiotics. Food in its natural state is food that is produced by the Lord and designed to nourish and build the body with nutrition. Food should not be confused with packaged, processed, canned, or boxed substances filled with synthetic chemicals, sweeteners, coloring agents, and preservatives that look like food.

Nourishing foods feed the body. Products that look like food can ward off hunger but cause a continual decline in the body. This is proven time and time again when we reverse the situation. More and more, we see the sick person who suffers from an autoimmune disease, chronic illness, exhaustion, or worse rebuild him or herself with real food and probiotics, and the illness gradually lessens until it no longer remains. Sadly, today we are seeing people who have multiple autoimmune diseases or struggle to make it through the day. They do not look sick; however, they suffer greatly every day. This is not optimal living. When we see these people switch food products for life building foods, which are nutrient dense, easy to digest, and building, we see recovery. This has been proven consistently and repetitively.

Food and probiotics are necessary for this process.

Just as not all foods are equally nourishing or necessary, not all probiotics are beneficial.

Choosing a probiotic today can be overwhelming. There are probiotic foods, probiotics online, probiotics in the coolers at the store, probiotics on the store shelf, probiotics at the local pharmacy, and probiotics in your refrigerator. Determining which one is best for your situation is no small adventure. Adding home-brewed probiotic foods only adds more confusion to the decision-making process. There are home-brews that use fancy jars and air lock containers and others that seek exotic ingredients. The thought of what to use for your specific situation can be daunting.

Some probiotics will put you in debt; others will feed the pathogenic bacteria you are trying to eliminate.

Every one of them is touted as the best thing for you, will save your life, will eliminate all your illnesses — according to their manufacturer.

Navigating these stormy waters takes knowledge, as well as trial and error. Using commercial probiotics or food probiotics can be a debilitating decision.

Choosing both may be best. The more studies that are run, the more we are finding the amazing powers of probiotic foods. Not only are their probiotic counts higher than commercial probiotics, but they have cofactors already in place assisting your body to absorb the benefits. However, some can do more harm than good.

Probiotics come in many forms. Some are over-the-counter wallet bleeders, while others can be made at home out of food. Food-based probiotics are favorable, because their probiotic strains grow naturally in their own ecosystem, which benefits the body perfectly. The probiotic market is not new. Probiotic foods have been used for centuries by almost all cultures. Probiotic foods are relatively new to America, in the general population.

The least expensive way to get probiotics is to home-brew them. It is also the best way to get the most probiotic content in your food, while knowing exactly what was added to the product.

The prefix pro- means "for," while the root -biotic means "life," making probiotic a benefit to the livelihood of your body.

When you eat probiotic foods, they feed the good strains in your body.

The good fights the bad, which then die. At this point they need to be eliminated, escorted out of the body. This keeps the body strong and helps it to fight infection, staying healthy. "Fermented foods are not optional," Dr. Natasha Campbell-McBride says.[i]

McBride is a trained Medical Doctor, Neurologist, and Neurosurgeon who is considered a pioneer in rebuilding a damaged microbiome. Her GAPS Protocol (*Gut and Psychology Syndrome*) has assisted millions of people on their path to repair.[ii]

Probiotics feed the good flora. The good fights the bad. Certain beneficial strains fight specific pathogenic strains. Using the strains correctly for your body can create healing at a faster pace.

Finding the probiotic that is the antithesis of the pathogen is the desired solution.

This area is still undergoing study; we have only scratched the surface. We do know that there are certain things that deplete our flora, while others build our flora.

Professor Eugene Chang works at the University of Chicago as a professor of medicine, specializing in gastroenterology. Chang told *Scientific American* that the speed at which our microbiome changes after the introduction of beneficial microbes is surprising. He said, "In contrast to what we thought might take days, weeks or years began to happen within hours."[iii]

Women who are prone to yeast infections, due to an abundance of pathogenic yeasts, can drink probiotic foods such as kefir, kombucha, or kraut juice and tell you that there is immediate change — even before they remove the glass from their lips.

Chang says that other factors are also affected by the introduction of beneficial microbes. He says they, "observed changes in the amount of bile acid secreted into the stomach and found that bacteria native to our food—microorganisms used to produce cheeses and cure meats—are surprisingly resilient, and colonize the gut along with species already in our microbiome."[iv]

Changing Your Bile Flow with Probiotics

Microbial Ecology in Health and Disease published a randomized, double-blind study searching to find "whether the ingestion of a fermented milk (FM) containing bifidobacteria and *L. acidophilus* could influence the metabolism of bile salts in the small bowel."[v]

Eight ileostomy patients were used in the study. These patients all had intestinal surgery on their small intestines during which their ileum was diverted to an opening in their intestinal wall for their gastrointestinal issues. Each person in the study received 100 grams of fermented milk with 107 CFU/g (colony forming units per gram) *Bifidobacterium sp.* and 108 CFU/g *Lactobacillus acidophilus*. The control group received the same fermented milk; however, it had been pasteurized, compromising the beneficial strains.

In the study, excreted waste was weighed and tested for bile salts for six hours after each meal.

They found that "free and secondary bile salts were significantly increased during the [fermented milk] period."[vi]

The *Journal of Applied Microbiology* says, "Certain intestinal microbes are known to produce vitamins and they are nonpathogenic, their metabolism is non-putrefactive, and their presence is correlated with a healthy intestinal flora. The metabolic end products of their growth are organic acids (lactic and acetic acids) that tend to lower the pH of the intestinal contents, creating conditions less desirable for harmful bacteria."[vii]

This means that if your pH is off, it will reflect pathogenic overgrowth in the bowel. Probiotics have been shown to change this back to normal levels.

They go on to say, "Normal microbial inhabitants of the GI tract also reinforce the barrier function of the intestinal lining, decreasing 'translocation' or passage of bacteria or antigens from the intestine into the blood stream. This function has been suggested to decrease infections and possibly allergic reactions to food antigens."[viii]

Each strain performs a function while they all work symbiotically as a team.

The journal further reported, "Lactic acid bacteria are known to release various enzymes and vitamins into the intestinal lumen. This exerts synergistic effects on digestion, alleviating symptoms of intestinal malabsorption, and produced lactic acid, which lowers the pH of the intestinal content and helps to inhibit the development of invasive pathogens such as *Salmonella spp.* or strains of *E. coli.*"[ix]

Probiotic use has been shown to assist digestion and to remediate hepatic encephalopathy, arthritis, inflammatory diseases such as IBS (Irritable Bowel Syndrome) and IBD (Inflammatory Bowel Disease), allergies, eczema, diarrhea, constipation, suppressed immune systems, hypertension, cancer, control cholesterol, yeast infections, bacterial vaginosis and even Helicobacter pylori infections, according to *The Journal of Applied Microbiology*.[x]

Individual Pathogenic Toxins Cause Specific Responses in the Body

It is no secret that autoimmunity comes from the health of the gut.

"All autoimmune diseases need to be treated by restoring and treating the gut flora," says Dr. McBride.[xi]

When the gut flora is dominated by pathogenic yeasts or bacteria and toxins, it responds according to what is present. Some pathogens release toxic gases such as ammonia, hydrogen gas, methane gas, acetone, ethanol, ammonia, and acetaldehyde, as well as 170 others.

"It's caused by protein and peptide complexes through the damaged gut wall. When these proteins absorb partially digested, the immune system finds them and says *you're not appropriate* and it starts developing antibodies against those proteins," Dr. McBride says. "A lot of proteins in our food are very similar to the proteins in our own bodies. These antibodies then find your own proteins in your body and start attacking those as well. This is called a mimicking phenomenon."[xii]

When the body is in attack mode against these pathogens, creating antibodies, it will develop disease where there are genetic weaknesses. When the toxins released by the pathogenic flora are absorbed into the blood stream, different things happen, depending on the person. For example, Streptococci living in the tonsils was the first marker for rheumatism.

McBride says, "They like to attach themselves to proteins and fats inside the body. That might happen in your joints. That might happen in your brain, or in your spine or anywhere else in your body. Once they attach themselves to that protein, they change its three-dimensional structure."[xiii]

When the immune system sees this changed structure, it recognizes it as foreign and attacks.

"It particularly happens with people who have a lot of Candida overgrowth who are generating a lot of acetaldehyde in their bodies. Acetaldehyde has an ability to attach itself to proteins in the body and change their structure," she says.[xiv]

People who suffer from heavy metal toxicity generally suffer from Candida in this state.

Signs and symptoms of Candida are frequent bloating, gas or general puffiness, a white layer across the tongue, frequent pink eye, red rash-like patches, hives, white crusty heals or feet, yellowed toenails, thick cracking toenails or fingernails that build up layer upon layer on themselves, foggy brain, athlete's foot, jock itch, vaginal yeast infections, fatigue, headaches, brain fog, dizziness, sinus infections, excitable energy, anger, irritability, fits, tantrum, giddy laughter for no reason, and even drunken behavior. Another sign is frequently occurring urinary tract infections.

The systematic name for acetaldehyde is ethanol.

The Environmental Protection Agency (EPA) says, "Acetaldehyde is mainly used as an intermediate in the synthesis of other chemicals. It is ubiquitous in the environment and may be formed in the body from the breakdown of ethanol."[xv]

In the body, when released by *Candida albicans,* it presents in different forms.

The EPA admits, "Acute (short-term) exposure to acetaldehyde results in effects including irritation of the eyes, skin, and respiratory tract. Symptoms of chronic (long-term) intoxication of acetaldehyde resemble those of alcoholism. Acetaldehyde is considered a probable human carcinogen (Group B2) based on inadequate human cancer studies and animal studies that have shown nasal tumors in rats and laryngeal tumors in hamsters."[xvi]

Most people aren't bothered by it, especially in low levels, as it makes them feel good.

PubChem, an open chemistry database at the National Institute of Health says, "It has a general narcotic action."[xvii]

They further add that it "causes irritation of mucous membranes."[xviii]

Removing chemicals from our food intake and eating nutrient-dense, inflammation-reducing foods in situations like this have been shown to help immensely.

For some people, taking out some of the pathogen feeding foods is enough; for others, being very meticulous with their food intake, as well as with specific rebuilding with proper probiotics is needed.

For others still, extreme measures need to be addressed. For example, a study reported in *Gut* says, "Translocation of *E. coli* across M-cells is reduced by soluble plant fibers, particularly plantain (weed) and broccoli, but increased by the emulsifier Polysorbate-80. These effects occur at relevant concentrations and may contribute to the impact of dietary factors on Crohn's disease parthenogenesis."[xix]

Specifically, they say, "Plantain and broccoli markedly reduced *E. coli* translocation across M-cells; apple and leek had no significant effect. Polysorbate-80 increased *E. coli* translocation 59-fold and, at higher concentrations, increased translocation across M-cells. Similarly, *E. coli* translocation across human Peyer's patches was reduced 45±7% by soluble plantain NSP (5 mg/ml) and increased 2-fold by polysorbate-80 (0.1% vol/vol)."[xx]

This means that eating broccoli and plantain assisted in repairing the microbiome. Polysorbate-80 did the opposite. The difference of broccoli and plantain weed on those with Crohn's Disease is remarkable. Take note that this is plantain weed, not plantain (the South American starchy banana that is often fried in butter and brown sugar).

Feeding the pathogens makes them stronger, while feeding the beneficial strains establishes homeostasis. While some of the pathogenic strains will always be with us, they have a function in the body at low levels. Eliminating these strains is impossible, as our bodies are designed to have these specific strains. When we die, *Candida albicans* is one of the key players that decompose our bodies. Keeping the pathogenic overgrowth under control is the goal.

Removing all sugars and keeping carbohydrates low are both important in assuring that the yeasts have no primary food source. Keeping a diet high in fat and low in carbohydrates, with specific fermented foods, is reported as the most successful treatment. Home-brewed kefir, yogurt, fermented garlic, and kraut juice are the champion yeast killers.

Pathogens and Picky Eaters

Bad bacterial overgrowth that develops into intestinal pathogens is being blamed for causing picky eaters to develop illnesses and autoimmune diseases. Dr. Natasha says, "Part of the toxicity has the structure of endorphins and opiates. When they hit the brain, they give the brain a pleasure signal. Many of them are similar in structure to morphine and heroin and other illicit substances. These children are addicts. The brain gets addicted to these chemicals."[xxi]

Dr. McBride says that these issues can all be resolved through sealing the gut, adding nutrient-dense foods, and rebuilding probiotics.

"Their gut flora is very abnormal. It's dominated by pathogenic bacteria, viruses, fungi, protozoa, worms, parasites, all sorts of things live inside their digestive system. As a result, the roots of their cells are sick, they're unhealthy. The person cannot digest and absorb their food properly, so they develop multiple nutritional deficiencies," Dr. Natasha says.[xxii]

She goes on to say, "The food gets digested and broken down by these pathogenic microbes and converted into thousands of very toxic poisonous substances, chemicals, which absorb into your bloodstream and get distributed around your body. Wherever they get to, they cause disease."[xxiii]

Pathogens in the intestinal tract damage the gut lining and cause holes, or ulcers, in the tract. Food no longer gets absorbed properly. Particles of food pass through these holes and are found floating around in the blood stream where food particles do not belong.

Picky eating is a sign of gut damage and an indication that the person is a perfect candidate for a gut healing protocol. The person craves the very foods that cause damage as the foods are feeding the microbes in the digestive tract. He or she is reliant on the foods that feed the microbes as they travel from the intestinal tract through the vagus nerve to the opiate receptors in the brain.

Processed, sugary, starchy, high carbohydrate foods are part of the root cause for the decline. Dr. Natasha discusses breakfast cereals saying, "These are the last thing anybody should be putting in their mouths."[xxiv]

Abnormal gut flora has signals, symptoms that tell us what is happening internally. One of the first signals is being a picky eater. These people often only eat a few foods and hold objections to textures.

"Treating any addict is difficult. They are often quite clever and manipulate. As soon as you turn your back to them, they'll undermine every effort," McBride says.[xxv]

The younger the child, the easier and faster the recovery. Often, the body wants the food it needs, but children trapped in a situation of addiction and gut damage usually stand their ground toward the opiate causing foods. These picky eaters pose a difficult situation, as they refuse to eat the foods that heal their systems.

If this is the case, Dr. Natasha recommends giving the child one teaspoon of the healing food, like meat stock; once the food has been taken by the child, a reward is given, along with an explosion of praise from both parents, including kissing, hugging, smiles, tickles and lots of praise.[xxvi]

Meat stock is not bone broth – a food which will not heal deeper damage in the microbiome.

Parents united are the most powerful and necessary force in this situation.

Repeat this process every five minutes. Eventually, the child will be drinking the essential meat stock. From there, add the proper healing foods one by one.[xxvii]

For difficult children who are older, the parent can motivate the child with something they want, such as a bike ride where the child leads, video games, a date with dad or mom, a hiking trip, camping, kayaking, paddle-boarding, a sleep over, frozen cookie sheets of ice in the bathtub to play Ice Road Truckers, a museum or park trip, etc. Activities outside are best, due to the healing aspects of the sun and nature itself.

"I'm absolutely convinced that every drug addict begins from abnormalities in their gut flora in their childhood getting trapped in this vicious cycle of cravings and dependency. Then it moves on to more serious substances than just sugars," Dr. Natasha says.[xxviii]

Dr. McBride emphasizes healing the body through animal protein and high-fat dairy, which nourish the body. Historically, all cultures except our current society have thrived well on animal proteins and high-fat dairy. Our current teachings heavily stress low-fat, processed foods and are not traditionally healthful. This happens at the same time that our society continues to get more ill.[xxix]

Dr. Natasha says, "Our immunity is made from half and half, protein and fat. The kind of protein the immune system is made from structurally comes from meat, fish, eggs and dairy. Plants have protein in them, but they have a very different amino acid composition."[xxx]

When the system is unhealthy, it is vital to nourish the body, so it can recover. "The building [and] feeding substances for the human body come from the animal foods, not from plants, because the animal foods are the easiest to digest, the easiest to assimilate. Their molecular composition of proteins and fats are very compatible with our own proteins and fats that the human body is made from."[xxxi]

The solution is to focus on the gut lining to reduce the toxicity, while feeding the beneficial bacteria. This is where probiotic foods and commercial probiotics are needed.

Rebuilding the Microbiome

Re-establishing a healthy microbiome comes from reducing inflammation and feeding the good guys that live in the gut. This can be done through eating probiotic foods, taking probiotic supplements, or doing both.

For centuries, people have been making probiotic foods to feed themselves. This develops a strong resistance to illness, as well as mental clarity and endurance.

Probiotic foods come in many forms and varieties. Picking the right one for you can be as simple as considering what sounds good to eat.

Different vegetables are available during different seasons. Preserving them by making them into a probiotic food helps to keep the nourishing food around, while also introducing healthy good flora to the microbiome throughout the year.

Taking commercial probiotics always involves variables uncontrollable to the consumer. In fact, you never really know what is in the product, as not all of the ingredients need to be listed. The supplement industry is a self-regulated industry, meaning that if they think something is appropriate for human consumption, whether it be a food product, coloring agent, ground up and processed wood, or other item, then it has the potential to become an additive in their supplements.

Chemicals, additives, and preservatives in food that are not specified on the ingredient list are common. The term "industry standard" can be a place to hide cheap, unhealthy ingredients in our food. An industry standard ingredient is one which is a standard ingredient among manufacturers of similar products when producing the product, and therefore not required to be specified on the ingredient list. It is a food ingredient hiding place.

For those of us with sensitivities, this poses a real problem, because there is no way of really knowing what is in the food.

Many examples of this exist; one is aluminum in American .cheese and processed cheese products. Adding aluminum to these forms of cheese is industry standard. If you have ever made homemade cheese, you have seen how it looks. It does not lay and fold like a piece of cloth. It has to be altered in some way for this to happen.

The *National Institute of Health, NIH,* considers the aluminum to be GRAS (Generally Recognized as Safe). Aluminum, in the form of sodium aluminum phosphate (SALP), is used for making the cheese smooth and uniform so that it is spreadable or able to be smoothed out into individually wrapped slices.

In spite of SALP being an ingredient in the cheese, it does not exist on the label, because it is standard in processing.

The NIH says, "Basic SALP is one of many 'emulsifying salts' added to process cheese, cheese food and cheese spread which react with and change the protein of cheese to produce a smooth, uniform film around each fat droplet to prevent separation and bleeding of fat from the cheese. This produces a soft texture, easy melting characteristics and desirable slicing properties."[xxxii]

The EPA says, "All processed cheeses may be enhanced with salt, artificial colorings, spices or flavorings, fruits, vegetables, and meats."[xxxiii]

This is standard processing procedure, *industry standard*; therefore, the process does not need to be added to the label.

Aluminum Sulfate is an industry standard ingredient used in canned crab meat, lobster, salmon, shrimp, tuna, pickles, and relishes.

Sodium Aluminum Sulfate is an industry standard ingredient used in pickles, relishes, baking powder and flour, including whole wheat flour.

Magnesium Aluminum Silicate is an industry standard ingredient used in chewing gum.

In the honey industry, it is an industry standard for the product not to be local honey made by bees. Instead, it is high fructose corn syrup with a small percentage of honey for flavor. It is cheaper this way. Many people who have life threatening honey allergies can readily eat mass produced store-bought honey because of the lack of actual honey in the product; however, they cannot touch local honey from a beekeeper.

Food Safety News says, "The FDA isn't checking honey sold here to see if it contains pollen." They say store honey is bleak, and that "U.S. groceries [are] flooded with Indian honey banned in Europe as unsafe because of contamination with antibiotics, heavy metal and a total lack of pollen."[xxxiv]

Fast food chain beef has industry standard fillers and additives "to enhance the flavor, texture and taste." Taco Bell was sued to change their "beef" labeling to "taco meat filling" because tests showed the beef content was less than 35% real beef. Taco Bell president Greg Creed said, "Our beef is 88 percent USDA inspected and not the 35 percent that's being claimed."[xxxv]

Shockingly, the USDA requires beef to contain 40 percent beef to be labeled as beef. This means a hamburger needs to be 40 percent beef, by weight, to be classified as beef.

The remaining percentage is made up of what is considered seasonings. These are isolated oat products and "other non-meat products used to add bulk and texture," like maltodextrin (corn based sugar), torula yeast (wood sugar), modified corn starch (a thickener using corn, wheat, potato, rice, or tapioca), soy lecithin (an emulsifier to hold the ingredients together), sodium phosphate (leavening agent salts), lactic acid (a pH regulator and preservative), caramel color, and cocoa powder (used as a flavor enhancer and color extender), and trehalose (sugar).

Hidden ingredients like these in food and supplements, including probiotic supplements, can feed the very pathogens we are trying to eliminate. Unknowingly, we could be feeding what we are trying to kill, and we are paying big money to do it.

Some of these ingredients are listed on the label, but others are not listed, due to industry standard protection. In addition to industry standard loopholes, regulation from the FDA appears to hover over product health claims more than over the ingredient list. Usually, investigations on health claims of products are preceded by a complaint, often made by a product competitor.

For this reason, many practitioners are big fans of probiotic foods over probiotic supplements.

Milk Kefir

Kefir is a fermented milk product used in many Slovakian and European countries. Some say that kefir making goes all the way back to biblical times when travelers would put fresh milk into skins (animal organs made into bags). The stomach and the bladder were both common skins. As the traveler moved across the land, the movement of the milk against the inside of the leather bags would cause a reaction.

This created kefir grains and kefir.

Kefir is highly popular for many reasons, mainly because it is such a strong probiotic. It is known as the champagne of milk.

Milk kefir proliferates with a plethora of *Bifidobacteria* strains; *Lactobacillus acidophilus, Lactobacillus Caucasus*; *Lactobacillus bulgaricus, Lactobacillus rhamnosus, Acetobacter* strains including *Acetobacter aceti* and *Acetobacter rasens*; *Saccharomyces boulardii* in three different strains (including *Saccharomyces cerevisiae* and *Saccharomyces unisporus*) *Candida kefyr, Lactobacillus kefiranofaciens, Lactobacillus paracasei ssp., Paracei, Lactobacillu delbrueckii, Lactobacillus plantarum, Lactobacillus kefiranofaciens, Lactobacillu kefiri, Geotrichum candidum*, and *Kluyveromyces marxianus*, just to name a few.[xxxvi]

Different factors affect the nutritional value of kefir, including the kind of milk, the milk fat present, the length of brew time, the yeasts in the air, and even what the animal ate before milking, as well as the season in which was milked. Some brews are said to contain 10 grams of protein per cup.

A University of Florida microbiology class studied the beneficial probiotics in kefir and came to some remarkable results. This data, added to previous findings on kefir, show the shocking probiotic count of kefir that has led many consumers to stop buying probiotics from stores, only to replace their probiotic with home-brewed kefir.

Monika Oli, professor of the microbiology class, is an avid kefir drinker and had her students test kefir from Glades Ridge Goat Dairy, owned by Greg Yurish. Preliminary results showed 10 billion colony forming units per milliliter.[xxxvii]

Oli is a Ph.D., Lecturer at the Department of Microbiology and Cell Science at the University of Florida; she researched with her students in a course module, "Read Your Microbiome – The New Gut Feeling," during the Fall 2015 module.

Ten billion colony forming units per milliliter is equal to 10 billion colony forming units per 0.03381 ounces. Since there are roughly 5 milliliters in one measured teaspoon, that makes 50 billion colony forming units per teaspoon, and 150 billion colony forming units per tablespoon. Home-brewed kefir, from raw milk, is proving to be a powerful probiotic.

Goat farmer Yurish says, "[The findings are] very interesting!"[xxxviii]

Professor Oli says, "We found 3 different strains of [beneficial] yeast and 5 strains of [beneficial] bacteria – all with quite different properties."[xxxix]

Oli says, "I am certainly an avid proponent of probiotics. I had my first kefir culture when I was 10 – growing up in Germany."[xl]

She hopes the findings will inform more pre-health students, as well as the general population, of the benefits of probiotics.

Further research showed the difference of colony forming units of home-brewed kefir in comparison to store-bought kefir.

Store brands are pasteurized after the fermentation process, altering the nutritional value. Third year University of Florida microbiology student Sylvia Stankov said, "A lot of those microbes aren't actually there, they're killed off in the process."[xli] Pasteurization is necessary for kefir to be transported and to sit on the store refrigerator shelf. If the product can continue brewing, it will bulge in the packaging or explode, due to fermentation pressure.

This pasteurization limits the spectrum of beneficial microbes, diminishing the whole point of eating probiotic foods.

Oli said, "I did an experiment with Lifeway, Publix brand and my own kefir and I found a 10 to the 7th difference in the live active cultures, a 10 billion bacteria difference between the store bought and homemade (made from raw goat's milk). If you buy the organic health brands they're a little bit better but they also have the sugars in them. The Lifeway had very little in it, by the thousand CFUs compared to 10 billion or so."[xlii]

Oli goes on to say, "We've [studied] yogurt many times before, commercial yogurt has barely nothing in it. Some are completely dead. It's basically useless to eat commercial yogurt."[xliii]

The microbiology class went further with their kefir studies and identified different strains along with the CFUs.

University of Florida pre-med student Beau Freedman said, "We performed serial dilutions from 10 to the negative 5th -10 to the negative 10th and we plated that on MRS and PDA (potato dextrose agar) plates for different bacteria and yeasts. We were able to isolate four different bacteria and three different yeasts just on those plates."[xliv]

He went on to say, "They each have their own health benefits, they all complement each other. We sent them off for sequencing after doing a PCR with doing a 16S for bacteria, 18S for the yeast. We found *Lactococcus lactis*, *Leuconostoc lactis*, *Enterococcus durans*, *Gluconobacter japonicus*, *Saccharomyces unisporus*, *Saccharomyces cerevisiae*, *Kluyveromyces marxianus*."[xlv]

University of Florida pre-med student Parker Novak said, "*Lactococcus lactis* is commonly used for fermentation."[xlvi]

Genome Research says, "*Lactococcus lactis* is a nonpathogenic AT-rich gram-positive bacterium closely related to the genus Streptococcus."[xlvii] This beneficial strain battling the pathogenic strain is why many researchers are pointing to kefir for reversing overgrowth of pathogenic Streptococcus, which is responsible for the recent rise in PANDAS (Pediatric Autoimmune Neuropsychiatric Disorders Associated with Streptococcal Infections).

Streptococcus is in the order Lactobacillales and in the phylum Firmicutes.

Firmicutes is considered the skinny strain. People who are strongly populated with Firmicutes are thinner than those who lack Firmicutes.

They go on to say, "A complete set of late competence genes is present, indicating the ability of *L. lactis* to undergo DNA transformation. Genomic sequence revealed new possibilities for fermentation pathways and for aerobic respiration. It also indicated a horizontal transfer of genetic information from Lactococcus to gram-negative enteric bacteria of *Salmonella-Escherichia* group."[xlviii]

Microbe of The Week, at the Missouri University of Science and Technology says, "The bacterium is also being looked at as a potential oral vaccine for developing countries against *Streptococcus pneumoniae*."[xlix]

Leuconostoc lactis is thought to form only from dairy origin. *The American Journal of Medical Sciences* says, "*L. lactis* colony morphology resembles a Streptococcus."[l]

Drowning Out Pathogenic Bacteria That Cause PANDAS Symptoms

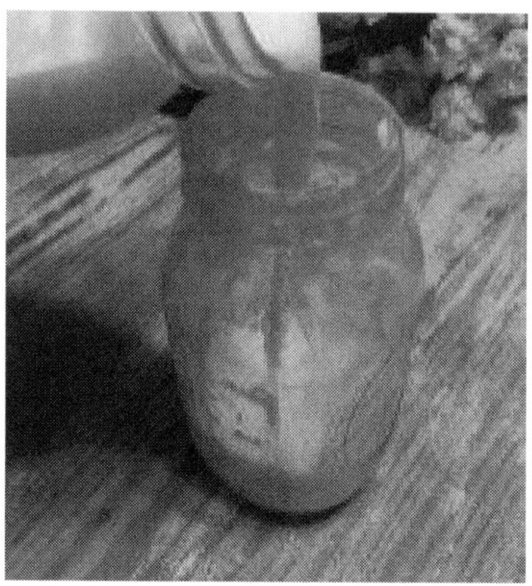

Beneficial strains of probiotics in kefir and other fermented milk products assist in drowning out the pathogenic strains in a PANDAS diagnosis. PANDAS was brought to light and named in the late 1990s by Susan Swedo, along with her colleagues from the National Institute of Mental Health.

Dr. Natasha says that PANDAS is a new title given to symptoms of a damaged microbiome that lacks the good bacteria to function properly. Rebuilding this microbiome is essential to homeostasis.[li]

The *National Institute of Health* says, "The diagnosis of PANDAS is a clinical diagnosis, which means that there are no lab tests that can diagnose PANDAS."[lii] They say that the development of tics and/or obsessive-compulsive disorders, with evidence of a prior strep infection (which, if unknown, can be determined through anti-*streptococcal* titers), points to PANDAS.

They go on to say, "The average grade-school student will have 2-3 strep throat infections each year."[liii]

Beneficial strains are known to drown out pathogenic strains. There are beneficial strains of streptococcus that are good for our bodies, as well as pathogenic streptococcus strains that give the PANDAS symptoms as well as many other symptoms. Mistakenly, many people avoid *streptococcus* strains at all costs, not realizing that the beneficial strep strains are the solution to the pathogenic ones.

Those with an abundance of pathogenic strains need to go very, very slowly. Too much can cause severe die-off.

The path to wellness includes drowning out the pathogens, no matter what the label of the disease is.

The *Bosnian Journal of Basic Medical Sciences* reported, "In the presence of probiotic strain the streptococcal adhesion [was] reduced, and this reduction was [not] significantly stronger if the probiotic strain was inoculated to the system before the oral bacteria."[liv]

Interestingly, there was a difference in the type of strain. They went on to say, "The *Lactobacillus acidophilus* had more effect on adherence of mutans streptococci than non mutans streptococci with significant difference. Adhesion reduction is likely due to bacterial interactions and colonization of adhesion sites with probiotic strain before the presence of Streptococci. Adhesion reduction can be an effective way on decreasing cariogenic potential of oral Streptococci."[lv]

These strains should be monitored to keep them in check. Overgrowth of different pathogenic strains leads to different diseases. For example, a cariogenic item causes tooth decay.

One study showed, "[*Streptococcus*] *thermophilus* may help balance Th1/Th2 responses. In one study, mice challenged with the antigenic protein ovalbumin produced significantly more TH1- associated IFN-gamma and significantly less TH2-associated IgE when fed milk fermented with *S. thermophilus* than when fed nonfermented milk."[lvi]

Another study shows that "mesenteric lymph nodes from colitis-prone mice orally with *S. thermophilus* and *B. breve* organisms displayed a cytokine secretory profile polarized towards a TH1 response. These studies suggest probiotic organisms like *S. thermophilus* may favorably influence immune function and provide therapeutic benefit in TH2-dominant conditions such as ASD (Autistic Spectrum Disorder)."[lvii]

Fermented milk products work together symbiotically. The *Czech Journal of Food Science* says, "Yoghurt production is the result of an arranged development of *Streptococcus thermophilus* and *Lactobacillus delbrueckii subsp. bulgaricus,* microorganisms that remain vital throughout the maintenance period."[lviii]

Current Opinion in Biotechnology says that fermented milks contain high levels of B vitamins like folate (B9) and riboflavin (B2), which are produced by the *Lactobacillus* and *Bifidobacteria* fermentation process. Some strains of Lactobacillus produce cobalamin (B12).[lix]

Using home-brewed kefir and yogurt together to rebuild the microbiome has been shown to be most effective. The University of Pretoria, South Africa says, "Probiotics strains and the traditional yogurt cultures, *Lactobacillus delbrueckii spp. bulgaricus and Streptococcus thermophilus* produce β-*Dgalactosidase*

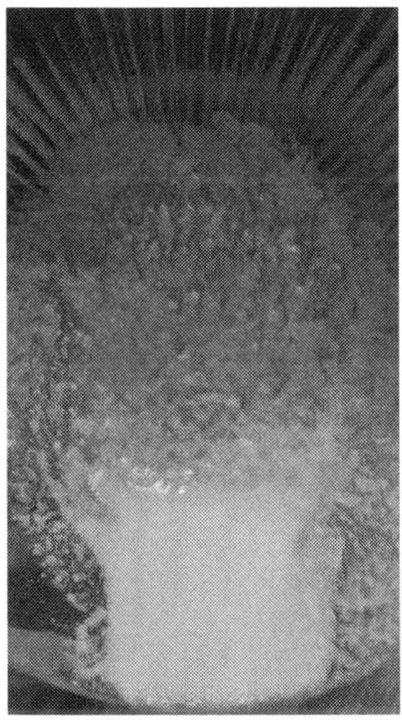

thereby improving tolerance to lactose. This is specifically done by rebuilding the missing bacteria and enzymes needed to digest lactose. The growth of *Streptococcus thermophilus* is, in fact, stimulated by amino acids and peptides produced by *Lactobacillus bulgaricus* from milk proteins."[lx]

In simple terms, they are saying that if you don't tolerate dairy, eating kefir will assist in rebuilding the foundation that assists in digesting dairy.

The Journal of Clinical Microbiology says, "*Leuconostoc lactis* is a streptococcus-like strain. Our *L. lactis* strains possibly represent a variant from those of a less versatile nature found in dairy products. Their low incidence in clinical material indicates that they are probably not normal inhabitants of humans, while in general the common isolation of Leuconostoc strains from meat products coupled with the divergent characteristics of our strains, indicates that the distribution of *L. lactis* outside dairy environments cannot be overestimated."[lxi]

Leuconostoc lactis and *Enterococcus durans* both fall under the same questionable category. They are thought to be pathogenic in the hospital setting; however, when found in fermented foods, they prove to be beneficial in rebuilding the microbiome. Research is still needed to determine the exact status and purpose of these strains that are still not fully known.

As previously stated, many species have good and bad strains. *E. coli* is the perfect example. Good *E. coli* assists in digesting lactose, the sugar in milk, while bad *E. coli* can send you to the hospital.

Enterococcus durans often presents a problem where it is identified incorrectly. "*E. durans* is not regarded as particularly pathogenic to humans and therefore VRE isolates of this species are not regarded as having the same significance for infection control as *E. faecalis* and *E. faecium*," says the *Journal of Antimicrobial Chemotherapy*.[lxii] Yet it is consistently found where repair is taking place, specifically as "DNA repair protein."[lxiii]

The Medical University of South Carolina BMC Microbiology reports that *Enterococcus durans* is a tyramine producer, an amino acid that "was found to be mediated by a transcription antitermination system, whereas the specific induction at acidic pH was regulated at transcription initiation level."[lxiv]

Critical Reviews in Biotechnology says, "The first step of acetic acid production is the conversion of ethanol from a carbohydrate carried out by yeasts, and the second step is the oxidation of ethanol to acetic acid."[lxv]

The amino acid tyrosine makes tyramine naturally in the body. For people with a damaged microbiome, these processes are potentially malfunctioning. Tyramine is responsible for blood pressure regulation.

For those who use natural foods to support their body, rebuilding amino acids assists in nourishment.

For those who rely on pharmaceuticals, this can be dangerous.

Monoamine oxidase inhibitors (MAOIs) block the enzyme monoamine oxidase, which is responsible for breaking down tyramine. Adding tyramine to a person's protocol when on MAOIs can cause issues with spiking blood pressure.

Ember Courtney, pre-dental major at The University of Florida, says during their microbiology study of kefir, "Sacromyaces was the yeast that we found. We found two different strains. It's generally used in most store-bought probiotics. We found *Enterococcus durans* stimulates gastrointestinal conditions and resists antibiotic damage. *K. marxianus* has been implicated in controlling the immune system by inducing pro-inflammatory responses which facilitates growth of Bifido bacteria [*sic*]."[lxvi]

Bifidobacteria should exist in dominant numbers in a healthy tract. As previously stated, stress is known to wipe out *Bifidobacteria*, leading to potential uprising of pathogenic strains. Many people can source their chronic illness back to a highly stressful situation in their life. The depletion of *Bifidobacteria* leaves the body susceptible to all sorts of uprisings.

Courtney stresses the importance of the synergistic effect of using multiple species at one time because they work collectively, impacting the microbiome. These are found naturally in probiotic foods.

Stankov, from the University of Florida, says, "We found a really interesting statistic for one of our yeasts – there are antibodies against this yeast found in 60-70 percent of patients with Crohn's Disease and in 10-15 percent of those with ulcerative colitis."[lxvii]

Professor Oli, from The University of Florida says, "One of the yeasts, clurglomysis is known to produce lactase so it breaks down lactose. Basically, kefir is naturally lactose free."[lxviii] The fermentation process eats up all the lactose.

S. cerevisiae, as reported by the research team, showed "positive effects on growth and production of Lactobacilli. *S. cerevisiae* has been used as a probiotic to treat bacteria-induced diarrhea."[lxix]

The researchers said, "We found prophylactic consumption of kefir can help with lactose intolerance. It's suggested in multiple sets that we looked at that people who have lactose intolerance consume kefir to build up a better tolerance to lactose."[lxx]

Since home-brewed kefir has eaten up the lactose in the milk, it becomes a tolerated dairy for those who are lactose intolerant.

Stankov goes on to say that consuming probiotic foods is rebuilding to a damaged microbiome. "You're reseeding what you have in your gut [, making it so that] whatever you eat you can digest. You get more vitamins."[lxxi]

Professor Oli questions the body's ability to retain the beneficial strains as the bacteria pass through your system. They are transient in nature, meaning they feed good bacteria as they pass through the tract.

She says, "It doesn't stay in your intestines. It depends on where you are in your gut health. If you have it regularly it doesn't matter if they stay or not because you're replenishing them." [lxxii] Continual consumption is recommended to maintain a healthy microbiome. This is not a one and done scenario.

The findings show that increased numbers of all species contribute to overall health. This means that if you are using milk kefir as a staple probiotic food, changing up the brew by adding some strawberries, vanilla, cherries, anise seed, or whatever you like to the second brew introduces different beneficial strains to the microbiome. Diversity is healthy, preventing dominant strains. The first brew is the initial fermentation where the kefir grains are put in the milk to brew for 24 to 27 hours. Afterward, the milk kefir is strained from the grains and added to another jar where the second brew flavors the milk kefir.

These findings show the reason that kefir is known for its enzymatic ability. It rebuilds the microbiome, specifically for those who have difficulty digesting lactose.

Some people with deeper damage in their intestinal tract cannot tolerate kefir. According to Dr. Natasha Campbell-McBride, this is due to the absence of enzymes that process the food.

For those who do not tolerate kefir, McBride recommends backing up to rebuild the missing enzymes needed to digest kefir.[lxxiii] For those with deeper damage in the microbiome, where the enzymes are few, the toothpick method can be used along with the dairy introduction schedule.

The dairy introduction starts with lots of animal fats, then proceeds to ghee, then grass-fed butter, then home brewed and strained whey, then yogurt (if diarrhea is present) or sour cream (if constipation is present), then milk kefir, then raw hard block cheese. For some, the toothpick method is used, if necessary.

The toothpick method means that you take a toothpick and just barely touch the food that is not tolerated, such as ghee on the dairy intro, and then touch your food. As this becomes tolerated, you put the toothpick deeper into the ghee and touch the food. As this is tolerated, you scrape the tiniest bit of the ghee and add it to your food. Once this is tolerated, you scrape up a larger amount, and then a larger amount, and so on, until you are tolerating a few tablespoons or more.

Intolerance to dairy does not mean that you will never eat it, but it does mean that you need to rebuild the enzymes that are missing so that it is tolerated. This is the function of the dairy introduction schedule.

The findings on health benefits of kefir are growing in number.

Osteoporosis International reported a study of 56 female rats, testing the effects of kefir and osteoporosis, specifically regarding calcium absorption. They say, "A 12-week treatment reduced the levels of C-terminal telopeptides of type I collagen (CTx), bone turnover markers, and trabecular separation."[lxxiv]

Trabecula are the supporting bundles of fibers that function as a mesh-work that creates the structure of bone.

They go on to say, "Treatment with kefir increased trabecular bone mineral density, bone volume, trabecular thickness, trabecular number, and the biomechanical properties (hardness and modulus) of the distal femur with a dose-dependent efficacy. In addition, in in vitro assay, we found that kefir increased intracellular calcium uptake."[lxxv]

Nutrition Journal studied natural milk antibodies versus pathogenic enteromicrobes and toxins with how they affect disease. They specifically researched the commensal bacteria in the gastrointestinal tract, with the aim of showing pathogenesis of rheumatoid arthritis (RA).[lxxvi]

The journal reports, "The natural milk antibody preparation containing high levels antibodies against pathogenic enteromicrobes and their toxins seems to be effective in a certain RA subset."[lxxvii]

In more detail, they say, "Based on our previous observations that milk antibodies may prevent the overgrowth of pathogenic bacteria and subsequently reduce the bacteria toxin production, we have studied the effect of milk antibodies on the disease activity in patients with RA. In the present study, we found that milk antibody treatment was associated with clinical improvement in 10 out of 18 patients with RA, which was uncontrollable by current therapeutics due to drug resistance, complications and risk factors."[lxxviii]

The Canadian Medical Association Journal reported in 1932, "Kefir is formed of a natural symbiosis of many yeast-like organisms, such as *Torula kephiri*, *Saccharomyces fragilis* and three kinds of lactic acid bacteria."[lxxix]

Kefir starter cultures have a remarkably high lactic acid bacteria count as well as high beneficial yeasts.

Adding whey protein to the mix of kefir fermentation has shown positive results. *The Journal of Dairy Science* has reported a study showing, "Addition of whey protein concentrate to broth stimulates the growth of lactic acid bacteria. The greatest growth in *Bifidobacterium lactis* was observed in milk supplemented with 2% whey protein concentrate."[lxxx]

Different factors affect brewing probiotics, including yeasts in the air and other fermenting products in the vicinity, such as kombucha or water kefir. Geographic location also affects the outcome of each brewed probiotic.

Many factors can change the probiotic findings in products like milk kefir. The grass the goat eats and where she is in her milking cycle are only two factors that affect the nutritional outcome. Goat milk has a different nutritional profile than cow milk, zebra milk, camel milk, or any other animal milk.

A review article, "Factors Affecting Goat Milk Production and Quality," in *Small Ruminant Research*, from researchers A.L. Goetsch. S.S. Zeng and T.A. Gipson, says that causes for differences in goat milk production include grazing and browsing vs. feed, confinement, plants available for consumption, forage impacting tissue mobilization, low body condition at kidding, and the number of milking sessions per day; all of these factors affect the quality and nutrition of the goat's milk.[lxxxi]

They go on to say, "As lactation advances after freshening, fat and protein levels decrease with increasing milk yield, and when production declines in mid to late lactation, fat and protein concentrations increase."[lxxxii]

This same quality, quantity, and timing is true for human breast milk.

The researchers further add, "The effect of milking frequency is greater in early and mid-lactation when yield is higher than in late lactation, along with a shorter period of peak production with one vs. two daily milkings. Effects of elevated levels of dietary fatty acids on specific long-chain fatty acids in milk and milk products vary with the fatty acid profile of fat sources used."[lxxxiii]

Many people use yogurt in their daily regimen for the probiotic benefits to their microbiome. Yogurt and kefir are considered cousins, related in their beneficial strains. Kefir is known as the champagne of milk, due to its bubbly effervescence and higher nutritional quality.

Kefir has a higher number of beneficial bacterial strains as well as beneficial yeasts when compared to yogurt.

As kefir is fermented, 10 to 20 different types of bacteria and yeast develop. The higher the quality of milk, the more the beneficial strains. Yogurt generally has just a few strains — more if the quality of milk is optimal.

Kefir is rich in the amino acid tryptophan, which is known for its relaxing impact on the body.

Advanced Biomedical Research reported a study testing the effect of kefir, evaluating its effects on anxiety, depression, and cognitive impairment.

The study sought a solution to the negative impact of nicotine withdrawal along with its mental and physical impairments. Nicotine is known to stimulate serotonin and dopamine levels, which are reward circuits in the brain. When this is removed, down regulation of the dopamine and serotonin levels negatively impacts the brain.[lxxxiv]

In the study, 48 adult male rats were purposefully administered nicotine salts to test the impact of kefir on the brain while going through nicotine withdrawal. Maze tests, as well as a forced swim test, were used to test anxiety levels, cognitive response, memory, and duration of physical ability.[lxxxv]

Remarkably, "there was a significant difference in their memory retention on the 6th day of training."

They concluded the same findings as other researchers, that kefir has been shown to prevent depression, anxiety, and cognitive abilities. However, they also discovered, "Kefir may be used as an available natural therapy for patients suffering from nicotine-induced anxiety and depression."[lxxxvi]

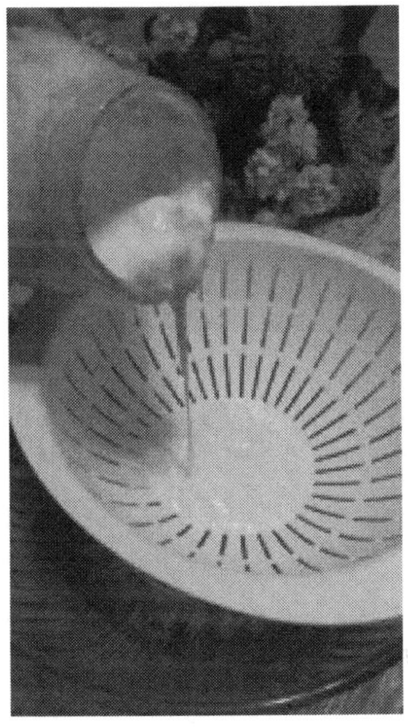

The *Journal of American Dietetic Association* confirmed what was previously discussed regarding digestion of milk for those who are intolerant. They reported a study done at The Ohio State University that showed that kefir improves lactose digestion as well as lactose tolerance, specifically in the 15 tested adults with lactose maldigestion.[lxxxvii]

These findings are not one-time, accidental discoveries. Many sources from many studies show the powerful nutrition of kefir.

Science Direct says that kefir contains the enzyme that digests lactose. They add, "Kefir is a good source of calcium, potassium and protein. But kefir also contains a wider array of microorganisms than yogurt does."[lxxxviii]

Steven Hertzler, a study co-author and an assistant professor of medical dietetics at OSU, says that kefir has many health claims including "enhancement of the immune system and improved digestive health, particularly with regard to lactose digestion."[lxxxix]

Breath hydrogen levels were reduced after drinking kefir. Hydrogen in the breath represents gas in the digestive track from pathogenic bacteria.

Mikrobiyoloji Bulteni, a Turkish microbiology bulletin says, "Bioactive peptides activate innate immunity by stimulating macrophages, increasing phagocytosis, augmenting NO and cytokine production and boosting the lumen levels of IgG and IgA+ B-lymphocytes."

They performed a study showing "the serum cytokine profiles of healthy volunteers after kefir consumption to evaluate helper T (TH) cell polarization and to bring out the effects on native and allergic immune responses."[xc]

Phagocytosis is the process where the good guys in the body surround the bad guys, bacteria or other material, and eat them up, dissolving them into themselves, and leaving the body free of potential pathogens.

They found that "results indicated that kefir use increased polarization of the immune response towards TH1 type and decreased TH2 type response and accordingly allergic response. The decrease in IL-8 level due to kefir use, might control the inflammatory response by suppressing neutrophil chemotaxis and activation."[xci]

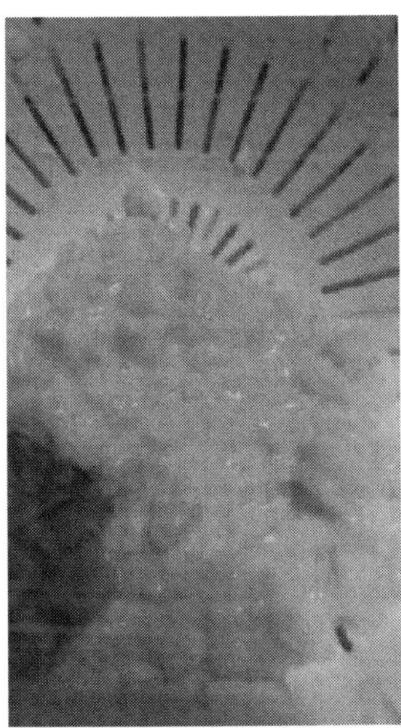

In the *Food Science and Technology Bulletin,* they say, "Many probiotic products have been formulated that contain small numbers of different bacteria. The microbiological and chemical composition of kefir indicates it is a much more complex probiotic as the large numbers of different bacteria and yeast found in it distinguishes it from other probiotic products."[xcii]

They go on to say, "At least one exopolysaccharide has been identified in kefir, although others may be present. Many bacteria found in kefir have been shown to have proteinase activity, and a large number of bioactive peptides has been found in kefir. Furthermore, there is evidence to show that kefir consumption not only affects digestion but also influences metabolism and immune function in humans."[xciii]

The Journal of Dairy Science reports on "kefir grains, which may contain up to 27 bacterial species from genera including lactobacilli, lactococci, leuconostocs, acetobacter, enterococci and micrococci and up to 30 different yeast species from genera such as kluvermyces and sacromyces; the strains are bound together by the exopolysaccharide kefira."[xciv]

These are several of the reasons that milk kefir is an integral part of GAPS healing.

Making kefir at home will always yield a higher probiotic count than buying kefir on the store shelf. This is because kefir can be made from the best raw milk or organic milk available and brewed for the full 24 hours or longer, yielding more beneficial bacteria and a reduced lactose content. Kefir grains look like gelatinous white cauliflower heads that start small and grow to the size of a marble or larger. They can explode and end up looking like a flattened burst balloon. The grains eat the lactose in the milk, meaning that the longer you brew kefir, the less lactose will be present. Generally, 24-27 hours is sufficient for removing nearly every bit of lactose. The ratio of grains to milk, temperature of your brewing area, and frequency of shaking your brewing jar (as kefir grains only brew what they are touching) all affect brewing time. A good ratio is one tablespoon of kefir grains to one cup of milk.

When the kefir brews, it appears like curds at the top of the jar. As the brewing process advances, the "curds" advance down the jar until they hit the bottom of the jar. The next step is a whey break line that appears like a line of clear, yellowish, or cloudy liquid, about a half of an inch from the bottom of the jar.

Most people like kefir best when it is pulled and strained for drinking just before the whey line breaks. Putting the kefir in the refrigerator slows the brewing process for consumption.

Kefir grains traditionally come from the Caucasus and propagate every time they are brewed, so once you get started, you'll be passing grains out to your friends.

To make kefir, pour your grains into a jar, cover them with milk, and allow them to brew with the lid on, directly on the counter top or in a cabinet until the whey line breaks. Again, usually one tablespoon of grains will brew one cup of milk in 24 hours; the more diluted the ratio is, the longer it will take.

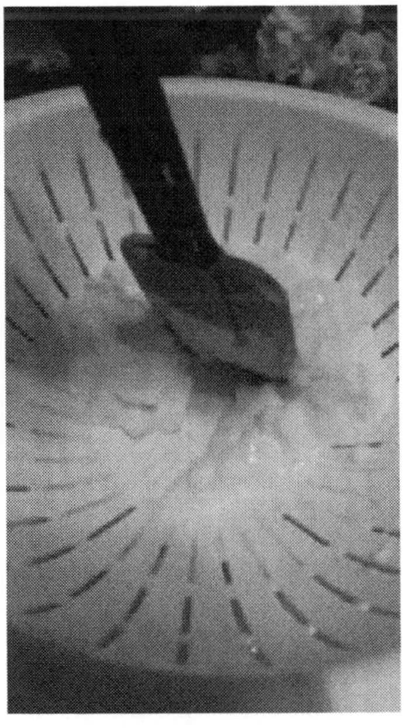

Be sure to shake your jar during the process to relocate the grains, establishing a more thorough brew. Strain your grains through a plastic, glass, or stainless-steel strainer, and drink the strained kefir. This can be used for smoothies, ice cream, cooking, or anything else you desire as a substitute for milk.

Temperature change, including heating and freezing grains, will negatively affect the probiotic count and productivity. Some kefir specialists say that freezing your grains is fine if you need to put them in long-term storage; others say that dehydrating them is appropriate. This is discussed further, below. Kefir grains may also be put in a jar with milk in the refrigerator, until you are ready to use them again. If you leave for vacation or do not drink your kefir as quickly as it is brewing, storing your kefir in cold storage, like the refrigerator, will slow the brewing process.

Grains are fine in the refrigerator for eight months, or longer, without using them. After two or three brews, they will perk back to life.

The vessel you brew your grains in will produce a better product and yield more grains if you do not wash it between brews. Most people wash their vessel when it begins to smell too sour at the lid.

Most kefir instructions say not to let the grains meet direct sunlight, come in contact with chlorine, be heated, be frozen, or come in contact with metal.

Pouring kefir grains down the drain is not recommended.

Eating kefir grains is fine, and even beneficial.

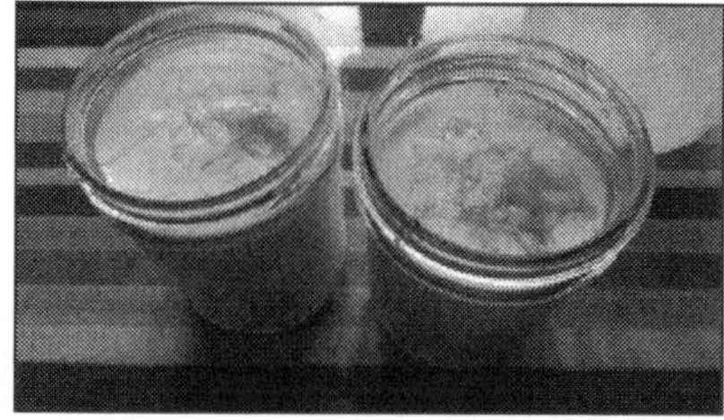

Making milk kefir is easier than it looks. As it is one of the strongest food-based probiotics, learning to make milk kefir at home will pay you back a million times more than the effort. The first step is to acquire kefir grains, which can be done online from Amazon or even Cultures for Health. Kefir grains look and feel like white, gelatinous mini-cauliflowers. As the grains grow, they can invert themselves, expand, and explode much like popcorn. This leaves a flatter, more stretched out kefir grain.

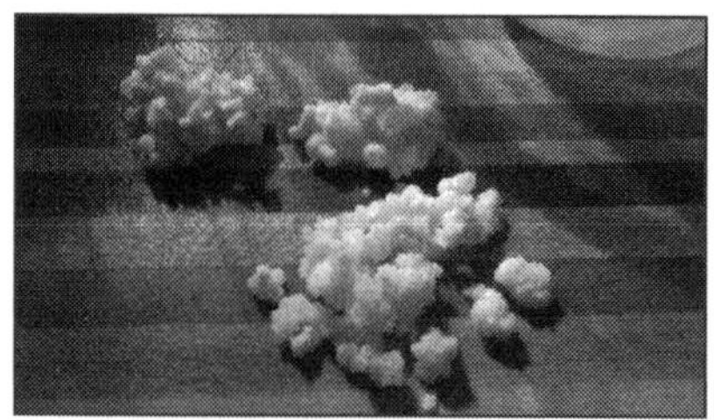

Put the kefir grains in a glass jar and cover them with milk, preferably raw milk. The general ratio of grains to milk is one tablespoon of grains per one cup of milk; however, this is not a solid rule. Fewer grains will still ferment the kefir; it will just be slower. More grains will ferment the milk into kefir faster. Put a lid on the kefir, as it is anaerobic. Fermenting milk kefir is not as concerning as fermenting vegetables in terms of keeping the grains submerged below the milk line.

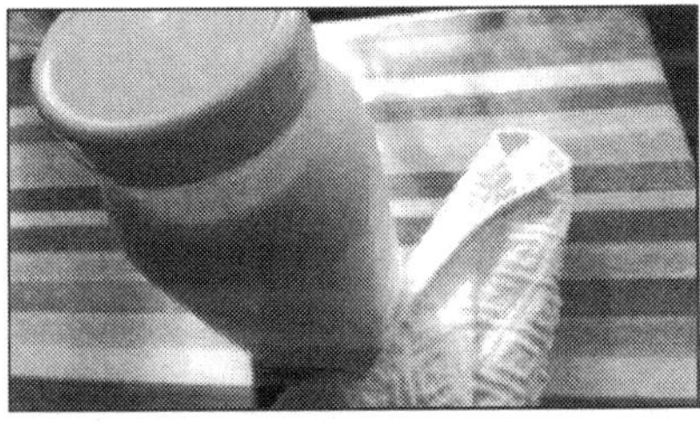

Shake the bottle once or twice throughout the day to relocate the grains. Kefir grains only ferment what they are touching, so relocating the grains will create a tastier, even-keeled product. When the milk is fully fermented, the lactose will be digested, the casein will be converted to paracasein, and it will be more solid in form, much like yogurt. As in the picture below, the kefir will stay in more of a solid shape. It can also be liquid, not thick, depending on what is happening in the milk and grains at the time; both are normal. Kefir is known as the Champagne of Milk, bubbly and effervescent.

As the kefir ferments longer, a whey break line will appear about two-thirds of the way down the jar. This means that all of the lactose has been digested and all the casein has been converted to paracasein. Most people like kefir best just before the whey break line breaks.

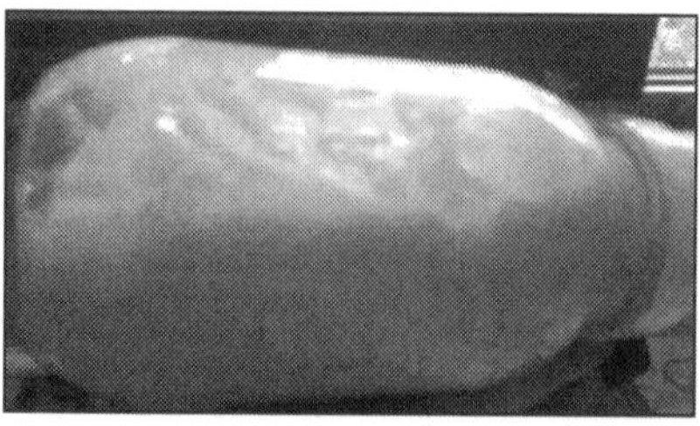

When you open the lid, the kefir will be thicker than milk and will stick to the sides of the jar. If it doesn't stick to the sides of the jar, it's fine. Every time you brew kefir, it will look a tiny bit different- sometimes more curd-like, other times more liquid.

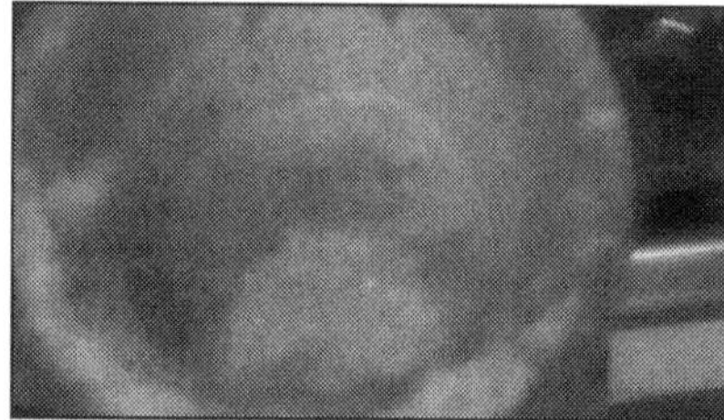

Use a stainless steel or plastic strainer, silicone spatula, and glass bowl. Place the strainer over the bowl, and pour the contents of the brewing milk kefir jar into the strainer.

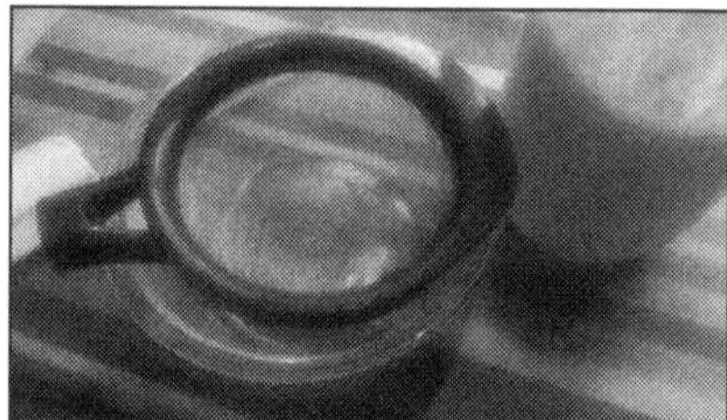

Push the milk back and forth. The fermented kefir will fall through the strainer, and the kefir grains will remain in the strainer.

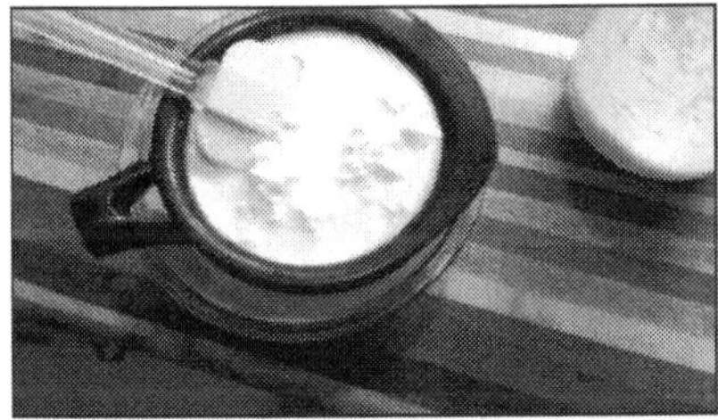

The more you brew milk kefir, the more the grains will multiply. Propagating grains are healthy grains.

They will all be different shapes and sizes, depending on their age.

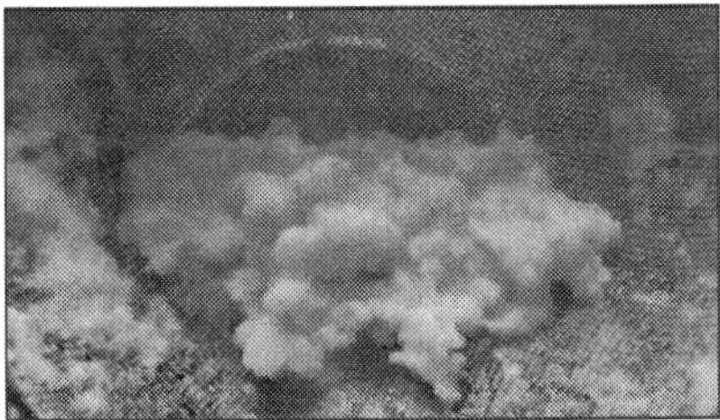

Put the kefir grains back in the same jar where they were previously brewed; there is no need to wash this jar every time you brew kefir. In fact, using the same jar will provide more grains, as the tiny dots stuck to the side wall are new grains forming. Some folks keep using the same jar until it smells sour on the top; then they switch to a clean jar. Pour new milk over the kefir grains. Put a lid on the jar, and let it sit another 24 hours.

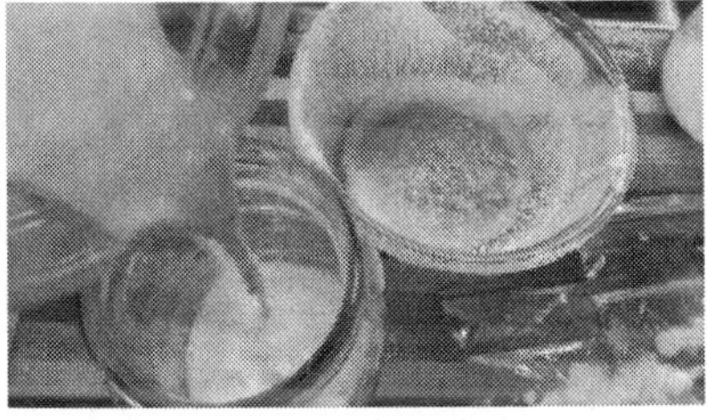

The milk kefir in the bowl is ready to drink. Many folks like it plain, while others like it mixed with vanilla and honey. A second ferment can be done using fruit. To do this, just pour the strained milk kefir into a new jar (without grains), and add fruit. Put a lid on the jar, and let it ferment longer, until the fruit has colored the milk kefir. The thinner you slice the fruit, the more completely digested it may be in the second ferment.

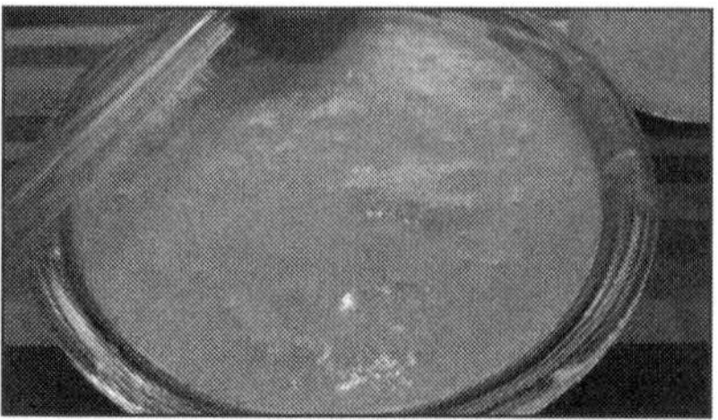

The brewing kefir can sit on the counter top or in a cabinet. There is a lot of forgiveness when making milk kefir. Some people just stick their hands in the jar to pull out the grains, then stick the grains in a new jar and pour new milk over the top, then drink the original jar of kefir.

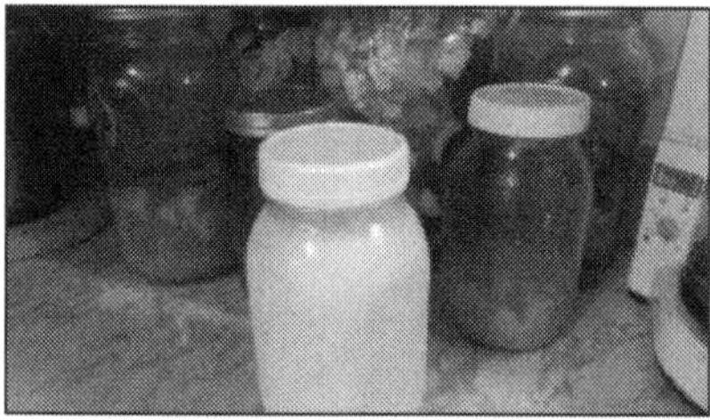

As your kefir grains make new baby kefir grains, you'll be overrun. They can be mailed to a friend by putting a tablespoon or two of grains in a double-bagged, snack-pack, zip-top bag, and then putting that in an envelope.

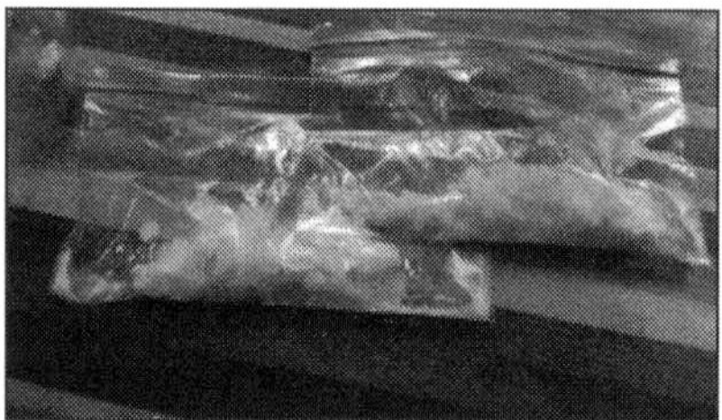

The more grains that are in the envelope, the more stamps you will need. Mailing them on a day that has consecutive mail delivery is best so that the grains don't sit in the heat or mail office for more days than necessary.

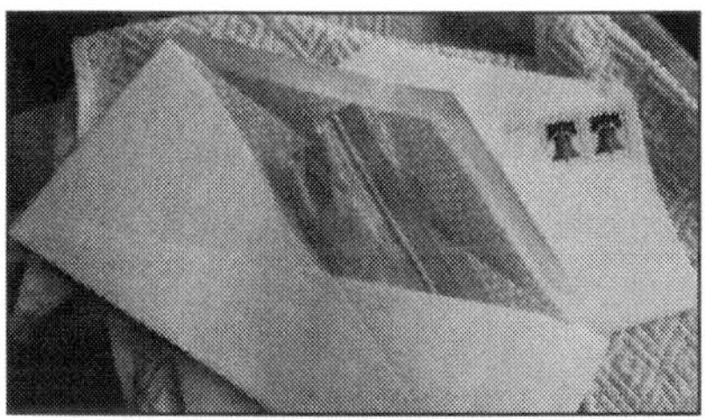

Milk kefir is specifically beneficial for drowning out pathogenic yeast strains, drowning out *Streptococcus* strains that cause tics, and drowning out pathogenic strains that cause eczema.

When the body has an overgrowth of yeast, these symptoms are possible. There are 250 yeasts in your body, one of which is *Candida albicans*. *C. albicans* is the most studied of the yeasts. Some researchers say there are 118 variable strains of C. albicans, while others say there are 187 strains. When they begin to thrive due to depleted beneficial strains, they change their shapes to meet their environment; they are opportunistic yeasts. These morphed yeasts take hold with strong tentacles and establish themselves in the microbiome in abundant numbers.

The best way to remove these pathogenic yeasts is to drown them out with beneficial strains, such as those found in milk kefir.

Fermenting Breast Milk

"Pediatricians found that microbes called *Bifidobacteria* were more common in the stools of breast-fed infants than bottle-fed ones. They argued that human milk must contain some substance that nourished the bacteria—something that later scientists called the bifidus factor," reported *The New Yorker*.[xcv]

This balance creates a healthy microbiome, a balance of the good and bad flora and bacteria. When this balance is not healthy, pathogenic flora blooms. This creates dysbiosis, an imbalance of the healthy microbes. Breast milk is probably the perfect food. Fermenting it amplifies its beneficial strains.

Some think that this is due to the over 200 human milk oligosaccharides known as H.M.O.s. These oligosaccharides are the third most abundant ingredient in human breast milk after lactose and fats.

The New Yorker says, "Richard Kuhn and Paul Gyorgy together confirmed that the mysterious bifidus factor and the milk oligosaccharides were one and the same—and that they nourished gut microbes."[xcvi] Kuhn is a chemist and Nobel laureate. Gyorgy is a pediatrician and breast milk advocate.

Bifidobacterium longum infantis, or *B. infantis*, is the most dominant microbe in the infant microbiome.

The New Yorker further states, "*B. infantis* digests H.M.O.s [and] releases short-chain fatty acids, which feed an infant's gut cells. Through direct contact, *B. infantis* also encourages gut cells to make adhesive proteins that seal the gaps between them, keeping microbes out of the bloodstream, and anti-inflammatory molecules that calibrate the immune system."[xcvii]

This information, combined with what we already know about fermented milk, leads us to believe fermented human breast milk to be an enormously beneficial super food. It proves to be very beneficial in those with great microbiome damage, like FPIES babies.

The Concerning Results of Freezing Kefir

To ship product without bulging and leaking packaging, a study was done freezing traditionally made kefir and commercially made kefir, counting the probiotic strains.

The study was performed as a Master Thesis for the Louisiana State University and Agricultural and Mechanical College, tested and written by Keely Virginia O'Brien. The findings were published in *The Journal of Dairy Science, The Official Journal of the American Dairy Association.*

In O'Brien's study, each variation of kefir was frozen directly after fermentation. The samples were thawed and plated, tested for *Lactobacilli*, *Lactococci*, and yeast. Thawed tests were done on day 0, day 7, day 14, and day 30.[xcviii] [xcix]

O'Brien says, "Commercial kefir products have been designed to reduce these effects by using a pure starter culture consisting of a mixture of bacteria and yeast species that give a flavor similar to traditional kefir, but some health benefits may be lost in commercial production due to reduced microbial diversity and lack of beneficial exopolysaccharides."[c]

In the study, the commercial kefir product tested was inoculated with a commercial kefir starter packet.

The traditionally brewed kefir was inoculated with kefir grains.[ci]

O'Brien found, "*Lactobacilli*, *lactococci* and yeasts were significantly reduced in number during frozen storage; however, the traditionally produced kefir was shown to have significantly higher counts of bacteria and yeast at each sampling."[cii]

This means the commercial starter packet that brewed the kefir left the probiotic food with a remarkably lower probiotic count than the kefir brewed with kefir grains.

After freezing, both products showed a reduction in probiotic strains as well as beneficial yeasts.

The kefir brewed with kefir grains showed higher beneficial bacteria and yeasts than the commercial starter packet kefir, but both were greatly reduced in their numbers in comparison to the unfrozen product.

O'Brien concluded, "Frozen storage and the development of frozen kefir products could eliminate most packaging concerns associated with the large scale manufacture of traditionally produced kefir, resulting in increased production and marketability of this healthful product."[ciii]

This happened, of course, because the product, after frozen, was greatly reduced in live activity.

O'Brien said, "Numerous studies have found [...] the total numbers of viable bacteria found in milk fermented with kefir grains to be greater than kefir made with isolated starter cultures (Marshall, et. al., 1985; Duitschaever, et. al., 1988; Marshall, 1993); this would [prove] advantageous during periods of cold storage, where the microbial counts are likely to be reduced. However, lactic acid bacteria has been shown to be remarkably stable during long periods of frozen storage; in a study by Lopez, et. al. (1998), lactic acid bacteria did not suffer any significant reduction in lactic acid bacteria during four months of storage at -23°C and retained a log count of around 107 cfu/g for the entire period."[civ]

To be clear, her study was attempting to prevent bulging and exploding packages while shipping them to the store. Her recommendation to use kefir from a starter packet is because there were fewer beneficial strains from a starter packet than from using kefir grains. When the reduced number of strains were further depleted, due to freezing, the product had less bulging and exploding. The containers survived during shipment. There was less product loss. Profit potential is higher with less product loss.

If the desire is to create the highest probiotic count possible, powdered starters and freezing are not recommended. These are best for continuing to make fermented milk products while traveling.

Using kefir grains, on the contrary, created a higher beneficial strain count, leaving a higher count after freezing, even though the count was greatly lowered by freezing.

Food Science and Technology Bulletin says, "Kefir grains themselves have inhibitory power against bacteria that can be preserved during lyophilization. Fresh kefir grains were found to inhibit the growth of the bacteria *Streptococcus aureus*, *Klebsiella pneumoniae* and *Escherichia coli*." [cv] Lyophilization is the process of freeze drying.

From these test study results, we see that there is a reduction of probiotic benefit when making popsicles out of a kefir. However, popsicles made with kefir still contain vast amounts of beneficial enzymes.

Optimal levels of probiotics should be achieved from non-frozen kefir; however, if the product is not tolerated at all, freezing it will make it less powerful and may be a way to strengthen weaknesses in the body.

This can easily steer folks away from making popsicles out of kefir; however, popsicles from kefir add beneficial enzymes and are a very healthy food and summer treat. Kefir popsicles are most definitely more beneficial that standard, store-bought popsicles.

Kefir popsicles can be made with berries, along with other fruits, and kefir. Anything can be added to popsicles in the same manner that anything can be added to smoothies. If the popsicle mixture does not taste good before being frozen, it will not taste good frozen as a popsicle.

Adding honey or dried fruit as a sweetener is not necessary.

Yogurt

Kefir's demurer cousin is yogurt, a dairy ferment with less overall probiotic, but a powerful ability to stop diarrhea.

The most well-known historical researchers who studied yogurt are Elie Metschnikoff, Director of the Institut Pateur, and his associates Leva, Pochon, Cohnenby, Herter, Brochet, and Lowbbel. The team studied the introduction of the bacteria in yogurt with both humans and animals.

The Canadian Medical Association Journal reported their findings, saying, "Professor Metschnikoff considered yogurt a natural and one of the most effective means of combating intestinal infections, intoxications, and putrefactions, which he thought were the cause of a great number of organic disturbances, such as premature senility, lack of vitality, poor colour and dryness of the skin, and arteriosclerosis."[cvi]

Metschnikoff believed that the Turks, Bulgarians, and Armenians lived healthy, vibrant lives due to their consistent yogurt consumption.[cvii]

His research of yogurt interested other bacteriologists, and the products increased on the store shelves.[cviii]

The *Canadian Medical Association Journal* said, "There appeared on the market a variety of pharmaceutical products, allegedly containing the ferments of yogurt and kefir, which met with varying success."[cix]

They further report, "In its genuine form it is prepared [through] the action of three kinds of bacteria – *S. thermophilus acidi lactici*, *B. bulgaricus*, and *Thermobacterium yoghourti*. The last the strongest of the three."[cx]

Many people avoid dairy and fermented dairy due to a casein allergy. Home-brewed yogurt (as well as other dairy ferments), when fermented for 24-27 hours, does not fall into this category; again, during the brewing process, casein is transformed into para-casein, albumoses, and peptones. The milk sugar is broken down into carbonic acid and lactic acid.

Yogurt has long been used medicinally in most ancient cultures. In 633 A.D. the most famous book of the time was published in Damascus. *The Great Explanation of the Power of Elements and Medicine* advises yogurt for dysentery and all inflammatory diseases connected to the stomach, liver, and intestines. The text reads, "Rid the body of poisons by destroying them."[cxi]

It further goes on to say, "[Fermented milk] strengthens the stomach, cures diarrhea, produces appetite, regulates the heat of the blood, purifies the humours, makes the blood more fluid, and gives a fresh and healthy colour to the skin, lips and mucous membranes."[cxii]

Julius Kleeberg reported with the Medical Clinic of the University of Frankfort, "In the use of yogurt and kefir we supply to the body one of the most perfect foods. It contains all the requisite nutritive elements in a form easily assimilable. These milks also have the notable advantage that they possess strong digestive properties even when the intestines are diseased."[cxiii]

The digestive properties are described as, "1) The chemical splitting of lactose; 2) the proteins of the milk are in part changed by bacterial action into albumoeos and peptones, which, besides being easy on assimilation are physiological stimulants of the hepatic and intestinal secretions; 3) a large quantity of lactic acid is produced."[cxiv]

Lactic acid is a digestive aid and works as an antiseptic in the digestive tract. A portion of alcohol and carbonic acid is produced, both of which stimulate the nerves of the tract.

"The influence of millions of powerful lactic acid bacilli, which corrects the abdominal flora and modifies the processes of and putrefaction, especially those that are dependent on the bacteria of the colon and the dysentery groups which can not develop in an acid medium," it says.[cxv]

Professor Baumgarten, a Professor of Bacteriology of the Bavarian Research Institute at Munich says, "With each gram of yoghurt are introduced into the body many hundreds of millions of living bacteria with demonstrated antiseptic power. [...] Treatment with yogurt is specially indicated in diseases of the digestive system associated with intestinal putrefaction, constipation, dysentery, tuberculosis and catarrh."[cxvi]

He goes on to say, "Yogurt is particularly beneficial in diseases produced by intoxication, in diabetes, rheumatism, furuneulosis, carbuncles."[cxvii]

It is important to note that the yogurt discussed here is European yogurt; it is not yogurt that is pasteurized, sweetened, highly processed, activated by powdered probiotics, and bought on American store shelves.

Home-brewed yogurt made from real milk would be comparable to the ones studied.

The most beneficial yogurt is made from unpasteurized milk sourced from a grass-fed, free-ranging, heritage breed animal that has not received any growth hormones, antibiotics or other medicines, or enhancing techniques.

According to Professor Oli's findings, "Commercial yogurt has barely [anything] in it. Some are completely dead. It's basically useless to eat commercial yogurt."[cxviii]

As with kefir, when yogurt brews, the casein converts to a paracasein, albumoses, and peptones, making the food digestible, even to those with a casein allergy. Nearly all see success with home brewed yogurt. If there is an issue, it is most likely die off as the good strains eliminate the pathogenic strains.

Researchers have been studying the specific strains in depth. They are finding that certain pathogenic strains cannot coexist in the bacterial ecosystem in milk ferments.

Researcher Kern "has demonstrated the inability of *B. coli* to develop in contact with yogurt. J. Cummata and U. Mitra, also, have shown that *B. typhosus, B. paratyphosus* and *B. diphtheria* lose their pathogenic properties if left a sufficient length of time in association with active yogurt cultures."[cxix] Again, this brings up the potential benefits of fermented dairy and its ability to fight off disease.

The journal continues to say, "Berthelot showed the same thing in connection with the coccus of cerebrospinal fever, as also did Rosenthal for the cholera vibrio."[cxx]

Sometimes, when scientists attempt to kill strains in the lab, they try to grow them also – or regrow them after drowning them out with beneficial strains.

This methodology is intriguing. It allows us to see what remains to be analyzed as viable or compromised.

The researcher reported to the *Canadian Medical Association Journal*, "I have seldom been able to recover pathogenic or saprophytic micro-organisms after they had been incorporated for two to four days with yogurt containing 1.65 to 2.00 per cent of lactic acid."[cxxi]

Applied and Environmental Microbiology reported a study that tested probiotic strains after probiotic yogurt had passed through the intestinal track. They found that "the ability to survive transit through the gastrointestinal tract, the ability to reach the distal tract in a viable form, and the ability to be recovered from feces by culture methods are unequivocally considered key features for a probiotic. We confirmed that yogurt bacteria, especially *L. delbrueckii subsp. bulgaricus*, can be retrieved from feces of healthy individuals after a few days of ingestion of commercial yogurt."[cxxii]

Milk Facts says, "The main [starter] cultures in yogurt are *Lactobacillus bulgaricus* and *Streptococcus thermophilus*. The function of the starter cultures is to ferment lactose (milk sugar) to produce lactic acid. The increase in lactic acid decreases pH and causes the milk to clot or form the soft gel that is characteristic of yogurt. The fermentation of lactose also produces the flavor compounds that are characteristic of yogurt. *Lactobacillus bulgaricus* and *Streptococcus thermophilus* are the only 2 cultures required by law (CFR) to be present in yogurt."[cxxiii]

Fermenting fresh milk from pastured cows, with a quality starter, is optimal and preferred. Choosing a farmer that you trust to supply your milk is important, but choosing a farm with a clean milking station is vital.

When making home-brewed yogurt, pasteurized milk should be heated up to 180 degrees, then cooled down to 120. At that point, stir in two teaspoons of a starter culture, and let it sit in your oven with only the light on. The starter culture can be from your previous batch of yogurt or from a quality yogurt from the store – preferably from grass-fed cows. It is optimal to let it sit in the dehydrator or yogurt maker at 110 degrees. If you are using fresh milk straight from the farmer, heating is not required, but stirring in more starter is preferred, as the good bacteria in fresh milk fight the starter. One ounce of starter per cup of milk is sufficient. GAPS people, or those who do not digest lactose, need to allow the ferment to brew for 24-27 hours so that all the lactose is digested.

In detail:

GAPS Approved Yogurt – A Probiotic Food

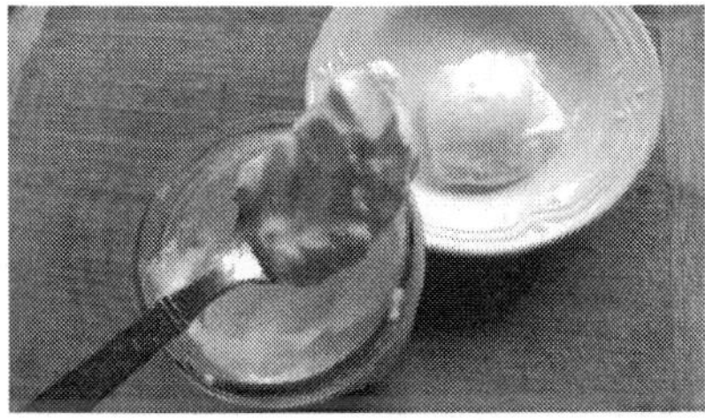

There are two ways to make GAPS compliant yogurt.

One method uses store-bought, organic milk; the other uses raw, unpasteurized milk.

When using store-bought, organic milk, heat the milk up to 180 degrees.

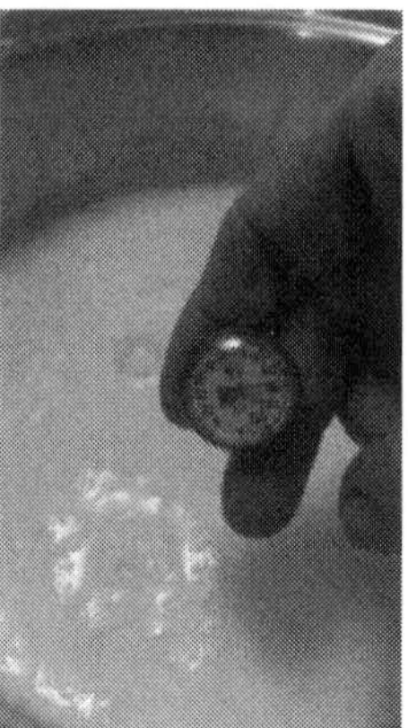

Cool it down to 120 degrees. If the milk is too hot, the starter culture will cook and be killed.

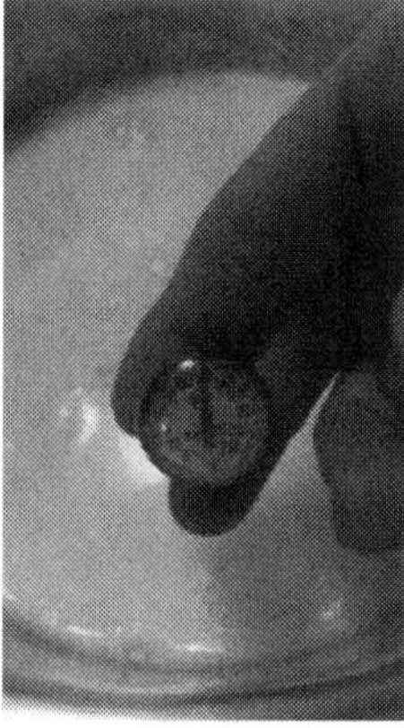

In a pint of raw milk, stir in two teaspoons of starter per gallon of milk. For a starter, use a quality, full-fat yogurt from the store, such as Nancy's, Seven Stars, White Mountain, Grass Milk, or Stonyfield, or use your previous batch of yogurt. Some yogurts are started with powdered culture and do not yield a good quality GAPS homemade yogurt. For this organic, store-bought milk variety of home-brewed yogurt, which has been heated and cooled, only the two teaspoons of starter per gallon are needed since the beneficial microbes are gone.

Whisk until combined thoroughly.

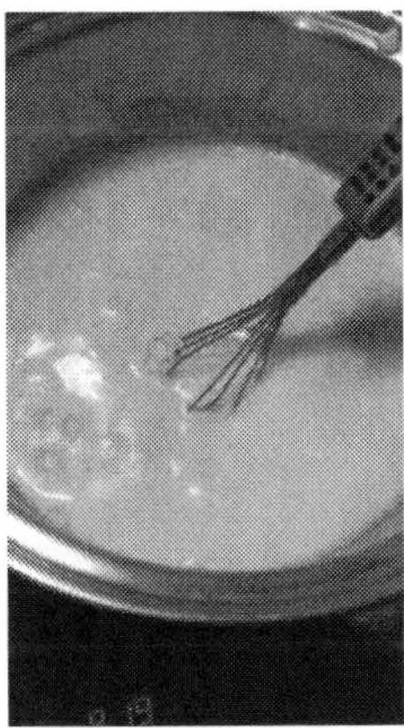

Pour the mixed milk mixture into Mason jars. Some prefer to put lids on the jars while they are fermenting, whereas others leave them off; the choice is individual.

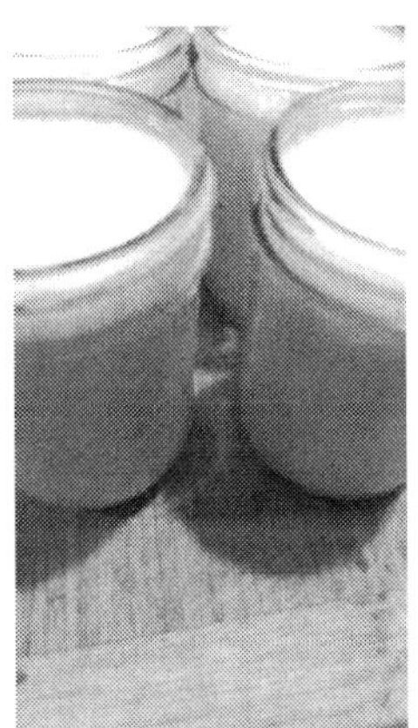

For making in an Instant Pot:

Put jars in Instant Pot, click on "yogurt," then immediately press "+" until the clock reads 24:00 or higher, until 27:00. If this button isn't pressed immediately, the machine will automatically default to an 8-hour yogurt brew. The machine will start itself. GAPS yogurt is left to ferment 24 to 27 hours, as this ensures that the lactose is consumed by the bacteria, leaving the yogurt lactose free. This brew time also ensures that the casein, the protein in milk, has been converted to paracasein, an easy to digest molecule. When fermenting in the Instant Pot, be sure the vent it open. If left closed, as it would be for pressure cooking, the yogurt will get too hot and create more whey than desired.

For making by other methods:

If you do not have an Instant Pot, put jars in the oven with the light on for the same 24-27 hours, on a heating pad with a towel over top of the jars, on top of an old refrigerator where heat emits, or in the dehydrator between 95- 110 degrees. Note: most dehydrators run roughly five degrees high, which will be too hot if the dehydrator is set at 110. Some folks ferment their yogurt successfully by putting an equal number of jars of milk with yogurt starter and lidded Mason jars filled with boiled water into a cooler or cooler bag for 24-27 hours.

***** If you are trying to make more whey, due to a dairy intolerance, where you wish to rebuild the precursor enzymes, set the dehydrator a bit higher. Temperatures at 115 degrees or just higher will yield more whey and less yogurt.

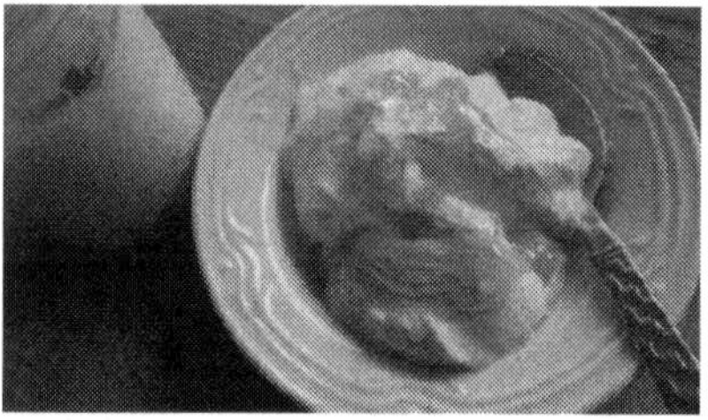

To make raw milk yogurt, put three heaping tablespoons of your yogurt starter or previous batch of yogurt into each pint Mason jar. Pour raw milk on top leaving an inch headroom. Stir the yogurt into the milk until thoroughly combined. Raw milk does not need to be heated prior to making yogurt. Raw milk yogurt requires more starter due to the high number of enzymes in the yogurt. The good in the milk fights the starter a bit, so more is required to get it started. Raw milk yogurt is teaming with more beneficial strains, as stated in the linked posts above.

Put jars in Instant Pot, click on "yogurt," then immediately press "+" until the clock reads 24:00 or higher, until 27:00. The machine will start itself. Again, be sure the vent is open. GAPS yogurt is left to ferment 24 to 27 hours, as this ensures that the lactose is consumed by the bacteria, leaving the yogurt lactose free. This brew time also ensures that the casein, the protein in milk, has been converted to paracasein, an easy to digest molecule.

If you do not have an Instant Pot, put jars in the oven with the light on for the same 24-17 hours, on a heating pad with a towel on top of the jars, or in the dehydrator between 95- 110 degrees.

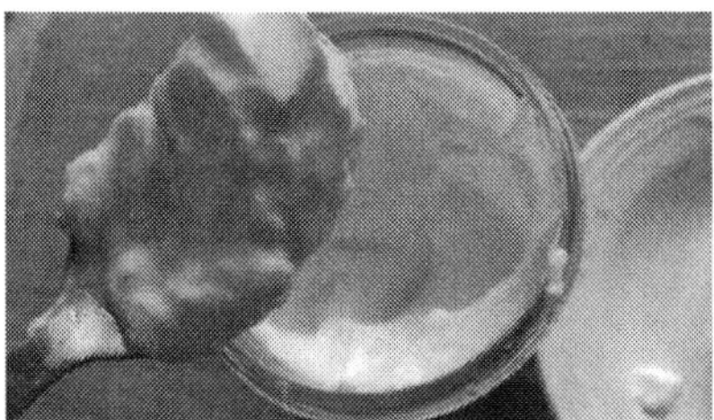

Some people add gelatin to their yogurt to make it thicker. Yogurt made with the proper amount of starter, after it is refrigerated, has the same consistency as the store-bought variety. Gelatin is not necessary. Adding gelatin instead of more starter robs you of a higher probiotic quantity in the yogurt. It is better to make the yogurt properly than to add other ingredients.

Therapeutic Advances in Gastroenterology says, "There are few controls on the labeling and quality of probiotic bacteria, thus care is needed in ensuring that the products used contain only the claimed probiotic bacteria, in the claimed numbers, and will deliver viable bacteria to the lower gut."[cxxiv]

The American Journal of Clinical Nutrition says that lactic acid bacteria digest the lactose in the milk. The result is *Streptococcus salivarius*, with subspecies of *thermophilus* and *Lactobacillus delbrueckii*, with further subspecies of *bulgaricus* containing individual species of *S. thermophilus, L bulgaricus, L acidophilus*, or *Bifidobacterium bifidus*. They reported, "All yogurts dramatically and similarly improved lactose digestion, regardless of their total or specific beta-gal activity. The response to fermented milks varied from marginal improvement with *B. bifidus* milk to nearly complete lactose digestion with *L. bulgaricus* milk."[cxxv]

Yogurt made from real (raw, exclusively grass-fed, unpasteurized) milk contains more probiotic strains than in pasteurized milk yogurt.

L. Acidophilus is of specific interest because it is acid resistant and bile salts tolerant, according to *IOSR Journal of Pharmacy*. They reported a study showing, "[…] lactic acid bacteria produce various compounds such as organic acids, diacetyl, hydrogen peroxide, and bacteriocins or bactericidal proteins."[cxxvi]

This is of utmost interest because of the increase in PANDAS with Streptococcal Infections. A study reported in the *Bosnian Journal of Basic Medical Sciences* said, "According to the results, it is clear that the presence of *Lactobacillus acidophilus DSM 20079* can cause reduction in the adherence of Streptococcal strains."[cxxvii]

Medline Plus says, "Lactobacillus is used for treating and preventing diarrhea, including infectious types, such as rotaviral diarrhea in children and traveler's diarrhea. It is also used to prevent and treat diarrhea associated with using antibiotics."[cxxviii]

Each family has different strains each strain performs a different job in the body. Lactobacillus is the perfect example. Some common names of strains within the Lactobacillus family are: *L. Acidophilus, L. Amylovorus, L. Brevis, L. Bulgaricus, L. Casei Immunitas, L. Casei, L. Crispatus, L. Delbrueckii, L. Fermentum,*

L. Gallinarum, L. Gasseri, L. Helveticus, L. Johnsonii, L. Lactis, L. Paracasei, L. Plantarum, L. Reuteri, L. Rhamnosus, L. Salivarius, L. Sporogenes.

Each strain has a benefit for the system.

Some people find it easier to take Lactobacillus supplements when they find they are deficient. Substituting these beneficial strains and other nutrients is often done through over-the-counter supplements. Reliability of this method is losing ground and showing such damaging effects that years later, patients are showing worse health after supplementation.

Two recent studies have been halted due to the negative results of supplementing.

"Supplementing isn't the same as getting nutrition from food itself," says Dr. Neal Barnard, MD, clinical researcher, president of the Physicians Committee for Responsible Medicine, Adjunct Associate Professor of Medicine at the George Washington University School of Medicine, and author of *Power Food to The Brain.*[cxxix]

In the Finnish study, 29,133 male smokers were used. In the U.S. study, 18,000 people were used, both male and female, including asbestos workers. The NIH reported that follow up continued for five to eight years with the "randomized, double-blind, placebo-controlled primary-prevention trial."

The NIH divulged the information, "Among the 876 new cases of lung cancer diagnosed during the trial, no reduction in incidence was observed among the men."[cxxx]

WebMD *Health News* reported that the trials were "testing whether beta-carotene and vitamin A could prevent lung cancer. Nearly everybody thought it would work. They were wrong. Lung cancer, heart disease, and death from all causes shot up in those who took high-dose beta-carotene."[cxxxi]

The outcome was shocking. "The people taking the beta carotene supplement ended up having more cancer than the ones taking a placebo," Dr. Barnard said.[cxxxii]

"Beta-carotene is one of just hundreds of carotenoids and if you're taking just one of them it might reduce the absorption of the others and it throws it all out of balance so you're worse off than if you hadn't been taking it at all," says Dr. Barnard.[cxxxiii]

WebMD *Health News* said, "Years after they stopped taking high-dose beta-carotene supplements, [the] group of smokers still suffer extra-high rates of lung cancer and death."[cxxxiv]

The New England Journal of Medicine reported the study, saying, "This trial raises the possibility that these supplements may actually have harmful as well as beneficial effects."[cxxxv]

When the placebo group was studied, it was uncovered that the test subjects were getting a lot of naturally found beta-carotene from foods, specifically vegetables. They found the same results to be true with Vitamin E.

Vitamin E in supplement form is missing cofactors, specifically the 8 forms of vitamin E found in almonds, walnuts, sesame seeds, and sunflower seeds.

Dr. Barnard says, "You're better off getting vitamins from food." He makes only one exception to that with vitamin B12, saying that B12 "is not made by animals or plants [;] it is made by bacteria. Meat eaters get B12 because the bacteria in a cow's intestinal tract will make it into the bloodstream and get stuck to the meat."[cxxxvi]

Certain brands of yogurt are another source of concern for Dr. Barnard, specifically for their probiotics. He says, "Those are just added with a shovel and a bucket in the factory. They're just an addition to the yogurt product. You can get any probiotic in a health food store."[cxxxvii]

Dr. Barnard says, "All the nutrition companies are pushing yogurt like crazy. It's a mistake. They should not be doing it."[cxxxviii]

The source of yogurt makes all the difference.

The PCRM (Physicians Committee for Responsible Medicine) awarded Dannon with the SICK award (Social Irresponsibility Towards Consumers and Kids) in 2013 saying, "Dannon is off the scale. It's high sugar, high calorie, it's basically selling ice cream or pudding and saying that it's somehow a healthy food. It's not."[cxxxix]

Dannon was sued for false advertising regarding their probiotic count in 2009. PCRM says, "They've had to pay out about $50 million in the past, so our feeling is the Dannon company has been taking it too far. They need to clean up their act."[cxl]

Real yogurts have live cultures. Live cultures grow from a starter culture where the product is left to culture at anywhere from 90-115 degrees for eight hours. Culturing the yogurt for 24-27 hours will ensure the near absence of lactose. Only a minuscule percentage of lactose intolerant people have issues with yogurt and kefir brewed this long.

Yogurt brewed at home from raw milk is a different category altogether. This is a whole food teaming with probiotic strains.

Synthetic supplements are often found with similar probiotic strains such as *Lactobacillus acidophilus*. When synthetic supplements are ingested, the body cannot process them like it can with whole nutrient-dense foods. The more damaged the person's microbiome is, the more they cannot process synthetic supplements. In fact, when the microbiome is damaged to the point of great inflammation and Intestinal Permeability, synthetic supplements usually cause great distress and erratic behaviors in the person.

The easiest way in which to acquire nutrients is through real whole foods, such as home-brewed yogurt.

Anaphylactic Allergies and Probiotics

Lactobacillus rhamnosus, a beneficial bacterium, combined with peanut protein, was accidentally found by Australian Murdoch Children's Research Institute to relieve peanut allergies.

The Journal of Allergy and Clinical Immunology reported an accidental finding with 62 children, looking to see if their intolerance would increase over an 18-month test period, adding peanut protein gradually to the mixture. "A double-blind, placebo-controlled randomized trial of the probiotic *Lactobacillus rhamnosus* CGMCC 1.3724 and peanut OIT (probiotic and peanut oral immunotherapy [PPOIT]) in children (1-10 years) with peanut allergy. The primary outcome was induction of sustained unresponsiveness 2 to 5 weeks after discontinuation of treatment. Secondary outcomes were desensitization, peanut skin prick test, and specific IgE and specific IgG4 measurements."[cxli]

Medical Daily reported, "Over 80 percent of the children who received the treatment were no longer severely allergic to peanuts by the end of the 18 months, when compared to four percent of the placebo group."[cxlii]

The NIH says, "There are qualitative and quantitative differences in the composition of gut microbiota between patients affected by FA (food allergy) and healthy infants. These findings prompted the concept that specific beneficial bacteria from the human intestinal microflora, designated probiotics, could restore intestinal homeostasis and prevent or alleviate allergy, at least in part by interacting with the intestinal immune cells."[cxliii]

They go on to say, "Lactobacilli and bifidobacteria are found more commonly in the composition of the intestinal microflora of non-allergic children and the enhanced presence of these probiotic bacteria in the intestinal microflora seems to correlate with protection against atopy."[cxliv]

Lactobacillus rhamnosus is a beneficial bacterium often used in probiotic strains of yogurt.

This study, with the potential threat of dangerous allergy symptoms, was performed with observant medical monitoring and should not be tried outside of proper medical care and observation.

Lactobacillus rhamnosus GR-1 adheres to the intestinal lining as well as the bladder and vaginal walls. Specifically, it combats the attachment of pathogenic yeasts. *L. rhamnosus* produces acid that kills viruses and attacks biofilms, but also is anti-inflammatory.

The Lawson Health Research Group at the Canadian Research and Development Centre for Probiotics, says, "*Lactobacillus rhamnosus* GR-1 was originally isolated in 1980 from the distal urethra of a healthy woman. *Lactobacillus reuteri* RC-14 was originally isolated in 1985 from the vagina of a healthy woman. It was first classified as *L. acidophilus* RC-14, then renamed as *Lactobacillus fermentum* RC-14. As the way that bacteria are classified changes with time, the strain was renamed *Lactobacillus reuteri* in recent years. All the publications with this organism RC-14, were performed on the same bacterium."[cxlv]

Lactobacillus reuteri RC-14 follows the same patterns. They go on to say, "It produces hydrogen peroxide that many believe is important in vaginal health. It also produces signaling factors that disarm toxins produced by *Staphylococcus aureus*, the bacterium that causes so many hospital infections and death (the superbug)."[cxlvi]

Administration of probiotics needs to be repetitive and deliberate in action, looking for die-off symptoms to be sure you are tackling weak strains. Probiotics do not remain in the body long term; they pass through (are transient), feeding the good bacteria and killing the bad in the process.

The British Journal of Nutrition reported a study showing that L. *rhamnosus* "induced weight loss in women was associated not only with significant reductions in fat mass and circulating leptin concentrations but also with the relative abundance of bacteria of the Lachnospiraceae family in feces.

The present study shows that the *Lactobacillus rhamnosus* CGMCC1.3724 formulation helps obese women to achieve sustainable weight loss."[cxlvii]

The American Journal of Clinical Nutrition says, "*L. rhamnosus* [is] usually associated with dairy products whereas *L. plantarum* is found in fermented foods of plant origin."[cxlviii]

Home-Brewed Sour Cream

The combination of quality, high fat dairy in the diet along with probiotic foods is proving powerful. High-fat dairy, in the form of sour cream, is considered the top choice for relieving constipation, while yogurt is for relieving diarrhea or loose stools. Some people need to exceed two cups of each to get the desired results.

If stool is not eliminated efficiently, bits and pieces will stick to the side walls of the tract. It will continue to grow as the years pass. For some, this can be problematic.

Fox News Health reported, "A 27-year-old man who was suffering from severe constipation for 10 years underwent surgery to remove a large stool from his colon."[cxlix]

The unidentified patient was evaluated at Second People's Hospital in Chengdu, China, after complaining of stomach pain, *Central European News (CEN)* reported. Although he had been admitted for the same pain previously, doctors had been unable to diagnose the cause.

A series of x-rays revealed that the patient's heart had shifted to the right because his colon had swelled to twice the normal size, *CEN* reported. Doctors diagnosed him with congenital megacolon, which can cause paralysis of the movements of the bowel and can sometimes lead to fecal tumors.

Surgeons later removed an 11-pound stool that had lodged itself in the patient's colon and caused his severe pain.

Sour cream made at home is associated with lubricating the bowel and keeping the stool moving.

Home-brewed sour cream is one of the healthiest home brews you can eat because it carries a negative charge.

"Sour cream is a very healthy food because it has both the fat and the lactate. Lactate is very, very interesting fuel because it's not sugar (and sugar has a lot of bad issues), and it carries a negative charge,"[cl] says Dr. Stephanie Seneff, the leading expert on sulfur and how it functions in the body.

Seneff is an electrical engineer, a computer science specialist, a biological scientist with a biology degree and food and nutrition specialty. She works as a Senior Research Scientist at the MIT Computer Science and Artificial Intelligence Laboratory.

Dr. Seneff adds, "It's very interesting that lactate carries the negative charge. Negative charge particles in the blood are very, very important to the blood's colloidal stability. This is a crucial thing that is happening to people as they get older — they lose the colloidal stability in the blood and they start to get into blood clots and hemorrhages."[cli]

Dr. Joseph Mercola refers to it this way: "It's kind of an electron deficiency syndrome."[clii]

The hardest thing about making your own sour cream is obtaining the raw cream. Organic cream from the store can be used, but it is not optimal.

To make home-brewed sour cream, use the same method as you would for home-brewed yogurt, but use cream instead of milk. Take one quart of raw cream, add 3-4 tablespoons of raw yogurt, and stir to combine them. Be sure to leave one inch of headroom (space on top of the cream between the cream and the lid). Put the lid on top and leave it on the counter for 2-3 days, shaking it twice a day. After you put the jar in the refrigerator, it will get even thicker. This can also be done in the dehydrator in the same way yogurt is made.

The Journal of Gastroenterology did a test during which they studied three groups of women: one group was fed a placebo; the second group was fed milk; the third group was fed fermented milk. After several weeks, they evaluated the women with functional MRIs while showing them a threatening, anxiety-producing photograph. The women who were fed the probiotic fermented milk had changed perceptions of the anxiety producing photograph in contrast to their prior response.[cliii]

The studies are consistent. At least from 2007 until 2015, studies have found that among other benefits, probiotics assist in relieving constipation.

For example, *The Internationale Journal of Pediatrics* reported a study with fermented milk because "inconsistent data exist about the role of probiotics in the treatment of constipated children."[cliv] Their goal was to determine the effectiveness of probiotics in childhood constipation, using a test group of 56 children, aged 4-12, who suffered from chronic constipation.

"Each sachet of Protexin was composed of seven probiotic bacteria including *Lactobacillus casei* PXN 37, *Lactobacillus rhamnosus* PXN 54, *Streptococcus thermophiles* PXN 66, *Bifidobacterium breve* PXN 25, *Lactobacillus acidophilus* PXN 35, *Bifidobacterium infantis* (child specific) PXN 27, and *Lactobacillus bulgaricus* PXN 39, TVC: 1 billion CFU TVC. [...]" they reported.[clv]

Fourteen males and ten females completed the study with this conclusion: "Our study showed that probiotics were significantly effective in improving the stool frequency and consistency in intervention group at the end of the 4th week."[clvi]

Other studies from *The Canadian Journal of Gastroenterology,*[clvii] [clviii] The *Iranian Journal of Pediatrics,*[clix] The *European Journal of Clinical Nutrition,*[clx] *Clinical Nutrition,*[clxi] [clxii] *World Journal of Gastroenterology,*[clxiii] [clxiv] *and The Journal of Research in Medical Sciences*[clxv] among others come to similar conclusions.

There are still reports that conclude that probiotics have little to no effect.

For example, *MedScape* reported, "Both probiotics and control group showed significant increase in stool frequency *versus* baseline. Probiotics did not increase stool frequency significantly *versus* control, and in fact at one point of time at week 2, control had significantly higher stool frequency compared with probiotics."[clxvi]

The secondary efficacy outcome was not remarkable, saying, "Compared with baseline, stool consistency improved significantly with probiotics but not with control. However, compared with control, the improvement in stool consistency with probiotic intake was not significant within the 4 week intervention. Magnitude of change in stool consistency, or effect size, was small but statistically significant in favor of probiotics."[clxvii]

The problem with their study may be that not all fermented probiotics are created equally; most are not worth the money.

The best results come from home-brewed raw dairy sourced from pastured cows that are exclusively grass-fed.

Yogurt Taffy, Sour Cream Taffy, and Kefir Taffy

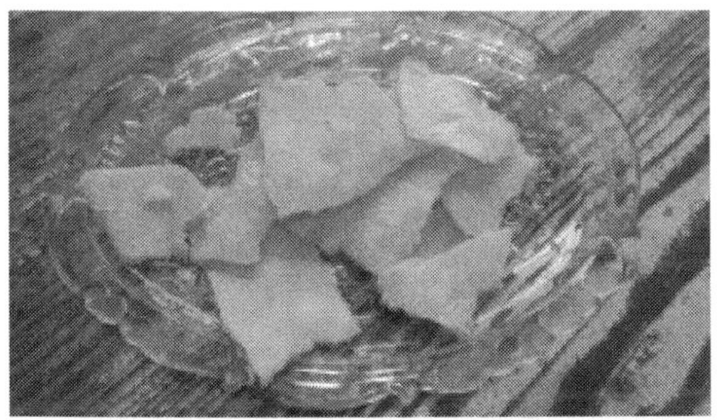

Yogurt taffy can be flavored with any fruit, local honey or dried fruits without added ingredients. This one is flavored with local honey as, in small amounts, it does not feed pathogens and is easily transportable.

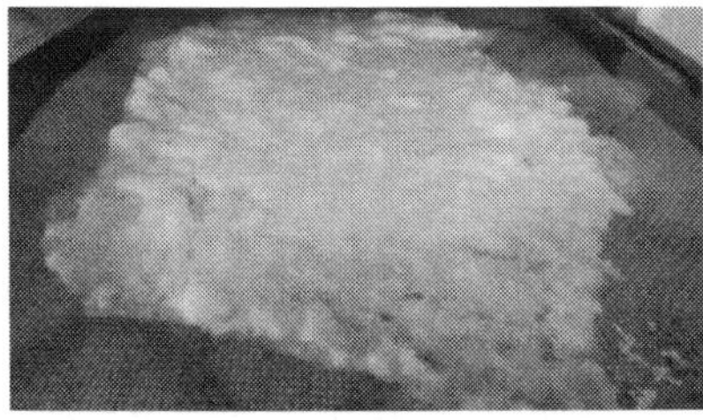

Spread yogurt on buttered parchment paper, preferably using home-brewed yogurt made from real milk. When it is dehydrated on parchment paper or wax paper that isn't buttered, it doesn't peel off; instead it becomes one with the paper.

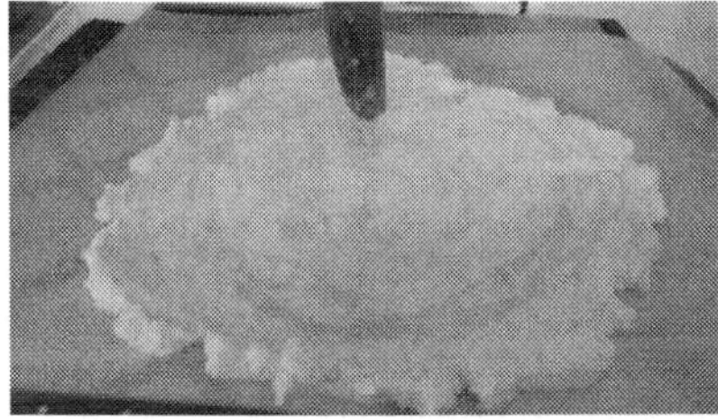

Yogurt taffy can be flavored with strawberries or drizzled with local honey or any other fruit and spice.

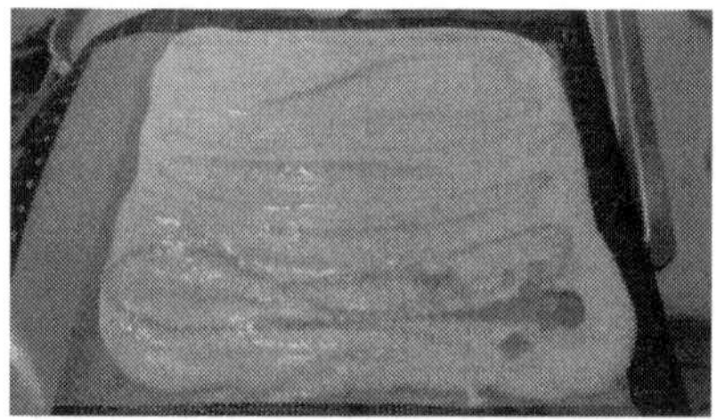

Dehydrate on trays until desired firmness at 115 degrees. Cut with kitchen scissors and store in snack pack bags.

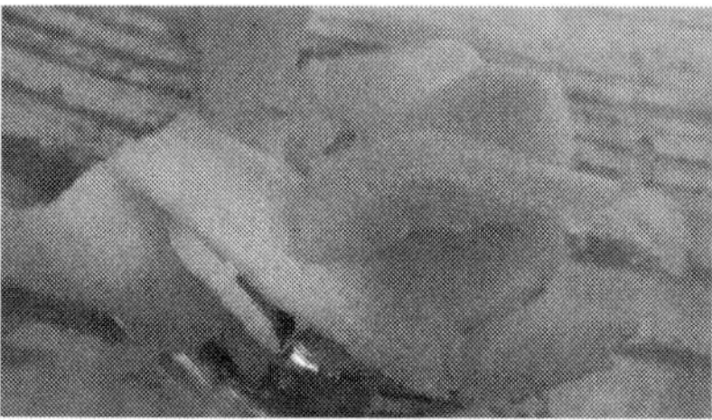

This works well as kefir taffy also.

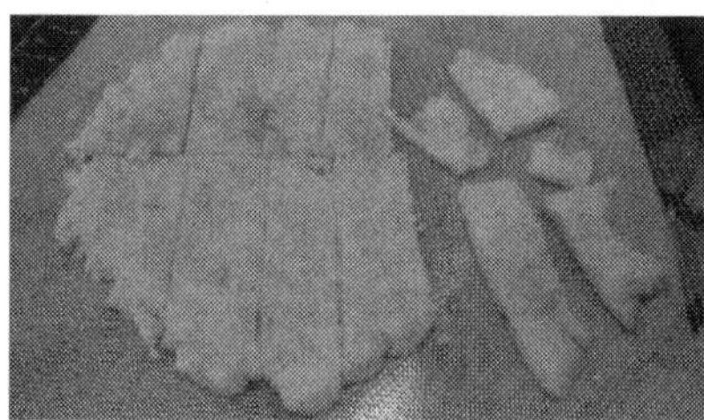

The thinner you spread the yogurt or kefir, the thinner and more cracked your taffy will be.

Sauerkraut

Sauerkraut tops the charts for probiotics, surpassing that of over-the-counter probiotics purchased.[clxviii]

Dr. Joseph Mercola sent his sauerkraut off to a lab and reported the findings of probiotics saying, "We had it analyzed. We found in a 4-6 ounce serving of the fermented vegetables there were literally ten trillion bacteria."[clxix]

That means that 2 ounces of home-fermented sauerkraut had more probiotics than a bottle of 100 count probiotic capsules. Translated, this means that a 16-ounce serving of sauerkraut is equal to 8 bottles of probiotics. However, 16 ounces of sauerkraut is not a serving.

He says that there are two ways a lab can analyze the microbial presence in the sauerkraut. "One is to measure the quantity of bacteria growing and then the more expensive process is to speciate the different types of bacteria."[clxx]

Dr. McBride says, "With every mouthful of sauerkraut, you're consuming billions of beneficial microbes which will be killing the pathogens in your gut, driving them out and replenishing the beneficial flora in your digestive tract."[clxxi]

As stated earlier with store-bought probiotics, the probiotic count of store-bought, shelf-stable sauerkraut does not compare to that of home-brewed sauerkraut. Sauerkraut in a sealed jar on the store shelf has been pasteurized, or flash-heated, to seal or secure the jar.

Heat kills the probiotic count.

Store-bought, refrigerated sauerkraut — kraut that has never been pasteurized — is a viable option but still not as good as homemade. Store managers are getting smart and putting glass jars of pasteurized sauerkraut with sealed lids in the refrigerator section to make people think they are probiotic products. Shoppers must be wary and educated on what they are buying. If a lid is sealed, the food inside is not alive.

If it has been pasteurized, it is not a probiotic food.

When kraut juice is introduced, people who have unbalanced gut flora with an overpopulation of pathogenic gut bacteria experience die-off symptoms such as diarrhea, rash, cold-like symptoms, flu-like symptoms, joint pain, headaches, irritation, anger, exhaustion, and many other. Many people can start with one teaspoon of sauerkraut juice, while looking for die-off symptoms, and gradually increase the amount daily or weekly depending on what the body can handle. The deeper the depth of damage in the gut is, the less an individual will be able to tolerate. Some people need to start with just one drop of sauerkraut juice, while others need to put one drop into a teaspoon or more of water, and take just one drop of that diluted version.

Remaining in a state of die-off is not recommended, as the body cannot heal in a state of inflammation. "If the gut is still damaged — if the gut flora is still abnormal — this river of toxicity continues flowing from the gut to the brain. Toxicity builds up again so the [person] slides back to whatever the disorder is," Dr. McBride says.[clxxii]

Nourishing foods feed the beneficial bacteria while starving out the bad bacteria. They drown out the pathogens.

Feeding the good through probiotics and cultured foods dominates the tract with healthy bacteria, making it impossible for pathogenic bacteria to thrive.

Since most probiotics on the market today are prophylactic, Dr. Natasha says that you should find "a really strong one made out of as many species of bacteria as possible."[clxxiii]

Cultured foods are foods that have been fermented, including sauerkraut, kimchi, kefir, yogurt, sour cream, kombucha, and water kefir, as well as other cultured foods. Fermentation preserves food. Sauerkraut is preserved cabbage that will last years and years in the refrigerator or in cool storage like a basement floor or root cellar.

If money is an issue and a patient cannot afford a good quality probiotic, relying solely on making one's own fermented foods is a perfectly viable solution.

To study autism and find potential cures, scientists bred mice lacking the Cntnap4 protein that links to autism. When the mice began to age and groom themselves, the scientists saw the pattern of mohawk hairstyles in the mice.

Live Science says, "The researchers engineered the mice to be missing a single gene, called CNTNAP2, which is thought to be involved in speech and language."[clxxiv]

HNGN, Headline and Global News, said, "Mice usually groom each other's fur. Over grooming is a 'repetitive motor behavior,' which could be a sign of autism. The finding marks the first time this type of behavior has been linked to a specific biological pathway."[clxxv]

Their grooming patterns follow a cycle of brushing their paw up their face to the top of their head. This formed mohawks in each of the mice in the test study.

The NYU Langone Medical Center released the news with the findings, saying that when they removed Cntnap4, GABA and dopamine were affected. Both are essential to the brain receiving messages from the body.[clxxvi]

Senior study investigator Gordon Fishell, PhD, the Julius Raynes Professor of Neuroscience and Physiology at NYU Langone, says, "Our research suggests that reversing the disease's effects in signaling pathways like GABA and dopamine are potential treatment options." Many people see positive results by adding GABA to their regimen.[clxxvii]

"GABA helps control impulses and regulate muscle tone while dopamine produces pleasant and soothing sensations. Repressing Cntnap4 led to a reduction in GABA and an increase in dopamine activity," says *HNGN*.[clxxviii]

WebMD says, "GABA is taken by mouth for relieving anxiety, improving mood, reducing symptoms of premenstrual syndrome (PMS), and treating attention deficit-hyperactivity disorder (ADHD). It is also used for promoting lean muscle growth, burning fat, stabilizing blood pressure, and relieving pain."

They go on to say, "GABA is used under the tongue for increasing the sense of well-being, relieving injuries, improving exercise tolerance, decreasing body fat, and increasing lean body weight."[clxxix]

The Denver Naturopathic Clinic says GABA is often used as a neurotranquilizer because "it inhibits nerve transmission in the brain, calming nervous activity."[clxxx]

They add, "The published research supporting any of these promotional claims is weak. Current medical opinion says that GABA taken as a supplement does not reach the brain and has no effect or benefit aside from being a benign placebo."[clxxxi]

The NYU Langone Medical Center says, "GABA acts in an inhibitory manner, tending to cause nerves to 'calm down.' Drugs in the benzodiazepine-receptor-agonist (BzRA) family (a family that includes true benzodiazepines such as Valium, as well as related drugs such as Ambien or Lunesta) exert their effect by facilitating the ability of GABA to bind to receptor sites in the brain. This in turn leads to relaxation, relief from anxiety, induction of sleep, and suppression of seizure-activity."[clxxxii]

They go on to say, "Unfortunately, when GABA is taken orally, GABA levels in the brain do not increase, presumably because the substance itself cannot pass the blood-brain barrier and enter the central nervous system. For this reason, oral GABA supplements cannot replicate the effect of tranquilizing drugs, even though they work through a GABA-related mechanism. GABA supplements can affect the peripheral nervous system, however, as well as any other part of the body not protected by the blood brain barrier. Some evidence suggests that orally ingested GABA might cause physiological changes that lead to benefit for hypertension."[clxxxiii]

Here's where it gets interesting!

Dr. Natasha Campbell-McBride promotes fermented vegetables like sauerkraut as well as home-brewed sour cream, yogurt, or kefir. She says that the role of home-brewed sauerkraut and high-fat dairy products is vital to recovery.[clxxxiv]

Specifically, Dr. Natasha says that Lactobacillus ferments prove to be highly successful with patients who suffer from autism, ADHD, and depression. These patients consistently lack Lactobacillus, a good bacterium that should be populating the gut flora to create a balanced microbiome.[clxxxv]

NYU Langone says, "Certain probiotics in the Lactobacillus family can be induced to produce GABA."[clxxxvi]

Dr. Natasha says, "The fact that your doctor doesn't know that something is curable doesn't mean that the knowledge doesn't exist elsewhere."[clxxxvii]

Psychology Today says, "Lactobacillus and Bifidobacterium species are known to produce GABA."[clxxxviii]

Making kraut at home is simple and easy. It is also one of the most economical ways to rebuild your immune system through probiotics.

Again, die-off symptoms are accompanied by inflammation. Healing and inflammation do not go hand in hand. It is important to keep inflammation down so that healing can take place; therefore, it is important to keep the amount of die-off down to just below a noticeable state. For most people, die-off is prevalent when eating sauerkraut.

Cabbage is high in anti-inflammatory properties and in vitamins A and C. Cabbage also reduces lipids in the bloodstream. When cabbage is fermented into sauerkraut, the fermentation process opens the cell walls, accessing a higher ratio of vitamins. It has been said that sauerkraut has 20 times more vitamin C than the head of cabbage before fermentation.

The African Journal of Science and Research said, "Healthy colons of humans contain some beneficial bacteria which feed on digestive wastes, thereby producing lactic acid. Without these beneficial bacteria, the digestive tracts become a thriving zone for pathogenic bacteria and yeasts, resulting in candidiasis. However, it is suggested that the consumption of lacto-fermented sauerkraut could help reestablish lactobacilli."[clxxxix]

Bacteria in your body outnumber your cells by about 10 to 1.

This means that approximately 90% of the body is made up of microbes.

In 1807, French psychiatrist Phillipe Pinel said, "The primary seat of insanity generally is in the region of the stomach and intestines."[cxc] Pinel is known as the father of modern psychiatry and came to this quote after working with mental patients for many years.

Sauerkraut is high in tyrosine, an amino acid that affects many aspects of the body, including blood pressure regulation and dopamine.

With billions of probiotics in each bite, sauerkraut is being ranked as one of the highest forms of probiotics you can eat, outranking over-the-counter probiotic pills, as previously explained. It is also one the easiest things to make in your kitchen, in which the chopping of the cabbage is literally the most difficult part.

First: Take a medium to large organic head of cabbage and chop it up as fine as you like. The finer the chop, the faster it ferments.

Second: Add 2 tablespoons of mineral salt and stir. You want to have all the salt equally distributed throughout the cabbage pieces. Some people go on to pound their cabbage with a cabbage pounder or a meat tenderizer; some even use the clean end of a baseball bat. Other people massage and squeeze it with their hands, while others just let it sit and allow the salt to break open the cell walls (this only works if the cabbage is chopped in the Vitamix or a similar machine so that the pieces are very small).

Either way, let it sit or pound it until the cabbage is limp and liquid has come out of the cabbage.

Letting the finely chopped cabbage sit is called salting.

If you have chopped your cabbage with a knife, the pieces will be larger, needing more pounding to open the cell walls.

All you really need to make sauerkraut is a bowl, a knife, cabbage, salt and a jar.

Third: Spoon the cabbage into Mason jars, packing it tightly so that there are no air pockets. Be sure that the top of the cabbage is covered by the liquid; this protects it from rising up and going moldy. Leave one inch of head space between the top of the cabbage and the lid. Brewing in a Mason jar is anaerobic fermentation — without oxygen. This only takes 4-12 days to brew. The warmer the temperature is, the faster it brews. If you need it to brew faster, use one of tablespoon salt and one tablespoon of whey.

Many people with deeper damage in their guts prefer kraut that has been brewed for 12 days or longer. Some do best with the ferment made last year or years ago. Once it is brewed to your taste preference, put it in the refrigerator to slow fermentation.

Take note — if any cabbage rises over the top of the water brine, it is fine. If it is left long enough that white mold forms, just scrape it off and eat what is beneath. This is kahm yeast, which is not a damaging mold to your body, says Sandor Katz, the Godfather of Fermentation and author of *Wild Fermentation*.[cxci] He says that if the mold does form, you should scrape off the white top before the layer gets too thick and reaches deep down into the jar; then put the jar in the refrigerator to slow down the fermentation process.[cxcii]

Since this is an anaerobic recipe, it is important to leave the lid on the jar; do not open it to see how it is doing. Go by the look of how limp the cabbage is; the lighter the color of the cabbage is, the more brewed it is.

If you just cannot stand waiting, then open it and taste it. Be aware, when you do, that you are letting oxygen in and halting the anaerobic environment, so it will take longer to brew once the lid is replaced. People do this, including Sandor Katz. You have not ruined it. If you prefer to taste your batch mid-brew, this is best done with a ferment that is fully submerged in brine, like when it is brewing in a fermentation crock — not when it is in a Mason jar.

There are literally millions of ways to make sauerkraut. The odds of doing it wrong are extremely low. Not making sauerkraut is probably the only wrong way to do sauerkraut. Each individual cook will make sauerkraut with a different twist — every one of them is correct.

RECIPE RECAP:

1 medium to large head of organic cabbage
2 tablespoons salt

Chop, salt, pack in jar, put the lid on, and leave on the counter for 4-12 days (preferably under a towel — it likes a dark spot).

The FDA has never found any incidents of someone getting ill or dying from sauerkraut or any other home-fermented vegetable. The process of lacto-fermentation contains a stage during the brew process that pathogens cannot survive. Pathogens like botulism, *E. coli*, and salmonella cannot exist in the second stage of the fermentation process.

Sauerkraut is famous for ranking high in *Lactobacillus*. When *Lactobacillus* goes in, *Lactobacillus* comes out, showing up in stool tests as high. This is not a matter for concern since the health of the person continues to thrive. Sometimes, chemistry in the lab shows different results from what happens in real life.

Lactobacillus probiotics secrete D-lactic acid.

"It's very confusing," Dr. Allison Siebecker, ND says. "D-Lactic acid, in and of itself as a real condition, is quite rare, but clinically I've been hearing about D-lactic Acidosis," she says.[cxciii]

Probiotics that contain *Lactobacillus*, like *Lactobacillus acidophilus*, secrete D-lactic acid. "In high amounts this has somewhat neurological consequences. Lactobacillus probiotics have been used as a treatment in D-Lactic Acidosis. The most prevalent bacteria that causes D-Lactic Acidosis is Enterococcus, so it's more likely to be an overgrowth of Enterococcus," she says.[cxciv]

Lactobacillus plantarum is found to effectively treat D-Lactic Acidosis, even though it secretes D Lactic Acid.

Soil-based organism bacteria probiotics and *Bifidobacteria*-based probiotics show benefits for these people because they are low in Lactobacillus.

Benefits of Sauerkraut

The intestinal tract is filled with good and bad bacteria that make up the microbiome. Feeding the good fights the bad. But… there is more to this! Some strains of bacteria make vitamins for our digestive system.

All probiotic strains are transient, meaning that they pass through the system instead of establishing colonies and remaining in the tract. Therefore, it is so important to eat commercial probiotics or fermented foods with every meal. Certain strains like soil-based organisms stay longer than others, setting up microbial colonies.

Lactobacilli and *Bifidobacteria* are human strains. These strains are abundantly found in a healthy tract. "They produce vitamin B12, B6, vitamin K2, biotin and other nutrients for us," says Dr. Natasha.[cxcv]

"Vitamin K2 produces almost identical benefits [to] vitamin D," Dr. Mercola told the American Nutrition Association.[cxcvi] The two work synergistically.

The highest producer of vitamin K2 is natto, a fermented soybean food that is known for being stinky and slimy.

The most common fermented foods are made with a cabbage base, fermenting into different versions of sauerkraut.

As the cabbage ferments, different things happen in each fermentation stage.

Susan Godfrey, from the Department of Biological Sciences at the University of Pittsburgh, studied microbial succession in fermenting cabbage and found that "the early drop in pH appears to constrain the growth of acid intolerant species[;] the more acid tolerant Leuconostoc are seen to bloom later, but fade subsequently because they are sensitive to the lactic acid that is their own fermentation product, and Lactobacillus appear to dominate at the end because they have the highest tolerance of the lactic acid they, too, produce."[cxcvii]

In Godfrey's study, they found that "even students sitting next to each other at the lab bench often isolate different organisms. Staphylococcus is usually found by at least one person in the class. No one student's data are exactly like anyone else's, since different sets of organisms are under investigation."[cxcviii]

The reason for this discrepancy is that each head of cabbage pulls different nutrients from the soil, is handled by different hands in the field, and is touched by different hands in the grocery store. The different vitamin structures and microbes that are present create different strains during testing.

As they studied the strains on the day the cabbage was placed in a 3 percent salt solution, they found:

Molds
Yeasts
Gram positive rods: *Bacillus spp, Corynebacterium spp., Arthrobacter spp.*
Gram positive cocci: *Micrococcus spp, Staphylococci* *
Gram negative rods: (facultative) *coliforms, Erwinia spp.*
Gram negative rods: (aerobic) *Pseudomonas spp.*

When they studied the strains the next day, day one of fermentation, they found:

Molds were gone
Yeasts
Gram positive rods: *Bacillus spp.*
Gram positive cocci: *Leuconostoc spp.*
Gram negative rods: (facultative) *coliforms, Erwinia spp.*

At day 4, when the samples were studied, they found:

Gram positive rods: *Lactobacillus spp.*

Gram positive cocci: *Leuconostoc spp.*

On day 7 and thereafter, they found:

Gram positive rods: *Lactobacillus spp.*[cxcix]

It is important to have all of the cabbage submerged under the brine while fermenting the cabbage. Exposure to air will cause oxidation, kahm yeast, and mold. Traditionally, for centuries, if mold occurred, it was scraped off and thrown into the compost bin while the rest of the ferment was eaten.

The American Society for Microbiology did a two-year study on commercial sauerkraut and found that "phages were very stable in such a low-pH environment. Each type of microorganism is involved in the microbial succession and contributes to the final characteristic properties of the fermented products."[cc]

When there is deep damage in the intestinal tract to the point of it affecting the histidine mast cells, which release histamine, adverse reactions to sauerkraut are often seen, unless the sauerkraut is fermented for an extended period – 3 weeks or longer.

Some people with severe histamine issues ferment their sauerkraut for 3 months or longer. The ascorbic acid, vitamin C, of the kraut consistently ranks high.

The Department of Biological and Agricultural Engineering at North Carolina State University built a fermenter to test the strains of bacteria as sauerkraut fermented. They found that "the 20 lactic acid bacteria isolates taken at the 28th day were all non-gas-forming rods, typical of *Lactobacillus plantarum*. Enterobacteriaceae were not detected during this stage."[cci]

Specific Probiotic Strains Have Been Shown to Boost Fertility

One of the first things we see with a decline in health is difficulty with conception.

Exposing the egg to *Lactobacillus crispatus* during in vitro fertilization ensured a higher likelihood of egg implantation, according to surgeon of vascular cancer, Leonard Smith, MD. "The likelihood that embryo can then be implanted and survive goes up. Bottom line, Lactobacillus on the egg helped in vitro fertilization success."[ccii]

Colonizing the vaginal area with the *Lactobacillus crispatus* proved beneficial.[cciii]

Since this is a strain in kraut juice, it leads us to believe that applying kraut juice topically, like you would lotion, may increase the chances of pregnancy. Topical application is best after getting out of the shower or bath, when the skin most absorbent.

Studies further showed that men who were put on probiotics to establish beneficial strains of bacteria in the gut showed a higher sperm count, a higher count of sertoli cells (which are responsible for testosterone levels), elevated testosterone, and more vigorous ejaculum.[cciv]

Dr. Smith said, "Mixed vaginoses that don't have a dominant strain do not seem to respond well to antibiotics. But guess what they do respond well to — probiotics and a probiotic diet. In addition to that, you can take fermented milk in a fermented solution of bacteria, instill it inter-vaginally, and switch them to a healthier vaginal profile, which needs to be done in the first trimester."[ccv]

He adds that an environment high in Lactobacillus showed less likelihood for a miscarriage or premature delivery. Group B strep was also knocked out with high applications of Lactobacillus. Dr. Smith recommends women to lubricate their feminine zones with Lactobacillus.[ccvi]

Group B strep left untreated could result in mental retardation or even death. Delivery room doctors do not really have a choice, legally; when a delivering mother tests positive for Group B strep, they have to administer antibiotics. Only 20% of cases are pathogenic and only 2% result in death.[ccvii]

PeerJ, a computer science publication says, "Evidence indicates that the intestinal microbiota regulates our physiology and metabolism."[ccviii]

PLoS One says, "We have found that the dietary supplementation of aged mice with the probiotic bacterium *Lactobacillus reuteri* makes them appear to be younger than their matched untreated sibling mice."[ccix]

The British Microbiology Research Journal studied Lactobacillus and fertility, specifically with *E. coli* strains, saying, "Upon mating and completion of gestation period 100% fertility was observed with 108 CFU (colony forming units)/20µl *plantarum* and 102 CFU/20µl *E. coli* (108 *colony forming units per 20 microliters plantarium and 102 colony forming units per 20 microliter E. coli. One microliter is one millionth of a liter*), whereas 100% females were infertile when administered with 106 CFU/20µl of *E. coli* along with 108 CFU/20µl *L. plantarum* and only 50% fertility outcome was observed with 104 CFU/20µl *E. coli*."[ccx]

Natural Fertility Info. says, "Many natural fertility experts agree; probiotic supplementation should be a part of regular protocol when treating infertility. Low gut flora gives rise to inflammatory disease. Endometriosis, PCOS (poly cystic ovarian disease), uterine fibroids, adenomyosis, dysmenorrhea (painful menstruation), Hashimoto's thyroiditis and autoimmune related infertility issues all have a common element involved: chronic inflammation. Inadequate levels of gut flora also give rise to the most common female vaginal problem: yeast infection."[ccxi]

Bioscience, Biotechnology, and Biochemistry reported a study on endometriosis in rats. They administered *Lactobacillus gasseri* and saw that "complete healing was observed in two of nine rats, but in none of the control group. These findings suggest that [*Lactobacillus gasseri*] is useful not only in therapy of pre-existing endometriosis but also in the prevention of the growth of endometrial tissue."[ccxii]

Two years prior, *Cytotechnology* conducted a different study of 66 people. "In this study, we evaluated the efficacy of *Lactobacillus gasseri* OLL2809 on endometriosis by the randomized, double-blind and placebo-controlled clinical study, especially against pain, which is one of the causative factors to decrease the quality of life. Results show that the tablet containing *L. gasseri* OLL2809 is effective on endometriosis, especially against menstrual pain and dysmenorrhea. Moreover, it was found that the tablet has no adverse effects. Therefore, it was suggested that the tablet containing *L. gasseri* OLL2809 contributes to improve the quality of life in the patients with endometriosis."[ccxiii]

PLoS One reported another study on male fertility regarding seminal fluid saying, "The analysis results showed seminal bacteria community types were highly associated with semen health. Lactobacillus might not only be a potential probiotic for semen quality maintenance, but also might be helpful in countering the negative influence of Prevotella and Pseudomonas. In this study, we investigated whole seminal bacterial communities and provided the most comprehensive analysis of the association between bacterial community and semen quality. The study significantly contributes to the current understanding of the etiology of male fertility."[ccxiv]

Smith says that it does help to take fermented foods and probiotics before and during pregnancy, and that they are not finding any studies showing that there is any danger.[ccxv]

Other clinical researchers in the field say that they have been seeing significant benefits for years from giving babies probiotics from fermented foods right from birth.[ccxvi]

Dr. Natasha says that women who lather their vaginal areas with home-brewed sour cream, yogurt, and kefir see amazing results with healthy children birthed through the canal. The beneficial probiotic strains creep up the vaginal canal and support the ecosystem with beneficial bacteria. Dr. Natasha says that this will benefit reoccurring UTIs or yeast issues, as well as benefiting the baby.[ccxvii]

Kimchi

Kimchi is a well-known probiotic food, traditional in Korean culture. The health benefits of kimchi are outstanding and should be part of a regular probiotic food regimen.

The Journal of Agriculture and Food Chemistry reported a study on kimchi showing its ability to degrade pesticides; it refers to "microorganisms in the degradation of the organophosphorus (OP) insecticide chlorpyrifos (CP) during kimchi fermentation. During the fermentation of kimchi, 30 mg L(-1) of CP was added and its stability assayed during fermentation. CP was degraded rapidly until day 3 (83.3%) and degraded completely by day 9."[ccxviii]

This means that as kimchi ferments, it degrades the pesticides to the point at which no pesticides are left on day 9.

The four CP-degrading bacteria in kimchi were all lactic acid bacteria strains: *Leuconostoc mesenteroides, Lactobacillus brevis, Lactobacillus plantarum, and Lactobacillus sakei.*

Critical Reviews in Food Science and Nutrition reported, "Numerous physiochemical and biological factors influence the fermentation, growth, and sequential appearance of principal microorganisms involved in the fermentation. The most important characteristics are the compositional changes of sugars and vitamins (especially ascorbic acid), formation and accumulation of organic acids."[ccxix]

The *American Society for Microbiology, Applied and Environmental Microbiology*, reported a 29-day fermentation study of kimchi. They found many species of Leuconostoc, Lactobacillus, and Weissella.

You can make kimchi from any vegetable. Koreans make kimchi from almost anything, including cucumbers, daikon radish, nappa cabbage, and even octopus. Generally, kimchi is made by fermenting Chinese cabbage with radish, red pepper powder, garlic, ginger, green onion, fermented seafood (jeotgal), and salts.

When they processed the kimchi at different stages, they found many different aspects, "It was also found a considerable amount of mannitol, a naturally occurring six-carbon polyol produced from the reduction of fructose by LAB in vegetable fermentations, accumulated during the fermentation. The presence of mannitol in foods results in a refreshing taste, and mannitol has noncariogenic properties and is a good replacement for sugars in diabetic foods."[ccxx]

Mannitol that is man-made is a sugar alcohol and is not processed by the body in those with a damaged microbiome. This is evidenced by those with severe gut damage, people considered "canaries in the coalmine." Others who have blood sugar troubles also respond negatively to sugar alcohols. For some, the negative response is not seen right away, but eventually, the body responds to sugar alcohols the same way it responds to sugar.

Microbial Cell Factories describes the benefits of kimchi, saying, "The advantages of acidic food fermentation are: (1) renders foods resistant to microbial spoilage and the development of food toxins, (2) makes foods less likely to transfer pathogenic microorganisms, (3) generally preserves foods between the time of harvest and consumption, (4) modifies the flavor of the original ingredients and often improves nutritional value."[ccxxi]

The Journal of Medicinal Food reported that kimchi assists in resolving asthma.[ccxxii]

They further reported a randomized clinical trial showing that kimchi improves serum lipid profiles in healthy young adults.[ccxxiii]

Kidney Research and Clinical Practice reported an "inverse association between kimchi intake and higher lipid levels in healthy and obese people."[ccxxiv]

Nutrition Research and Practice reported a large study on rats and found that "after 2 weeks of kimchi supplementation, the [blood pressures of the] group were significantly lower."[ccxxv]

Nutritional Research reported a study which hypothesized that "consumption of fermented kimchi would have more beneficial effects compared with that of fresh kimchi on metabolic parameters that are related to cardiovascular disease and metabolic syndrome risks in overweight and obese subjects."

What they found was that "anthropometric data showed significant decreases in body weight, body mass index, and body fat in both groups, and the fermented kimchi group showed a significant decrease in the waist-hip ratio and fasting blood glucose. Net differences in the systolic blood pressure, diastolic blood pressure, percent body fat, fasting glucose, and total cholesterol in the fermented kimchi group were significantly greater than those in the fresh kimchi group."[ccxxvi]

They concluded, "Ingestion of fermented kimchi had positive effects on various factors associated with metabolic syndrome, including systolic and diastolic blood pressures, percent body fat, fasting glucose, and total cholesterol, compared with the fresh kimchi."[ccxxvii]

Chef Judy Joo told *Fox News*, "Koreans don't feel that they've really eaten until they've had kimchi."

They go on to say, "The longer kimchi ferments, the greater the health benefit."[ccxxviii]

There are many ways to make each individual food, including kimchi. As a traditional food, sourced from one country alone, this is the perfect example of variety in making the product.

Some recipes call for nappa cabbage, carrots, ginger, garlic, and whey, while others add fish sauce and red pepper flakes. Even Koreans make kimchi differently from other Koreans. Some add three to four containers of canned anchovies, including the olive oil, in addition to fish sauce and a pear. Others bring flour and water to a boil, cool it down, then bring it to a boil again, and pour it over the vegetable mixture. They say that the starch is absolutely needed in the kimchi; however, others simply use the salt and vegetable with great results.

Some ferment their product in clay pots buried in the ground; others use plastic tubs; while others use glass jars.

There is no wrong way to make kimchi. Each person, and each batch, will produce a different outcome. The only wrong thing is not making it at all. This is the case for every ferment.

Kraut Juice

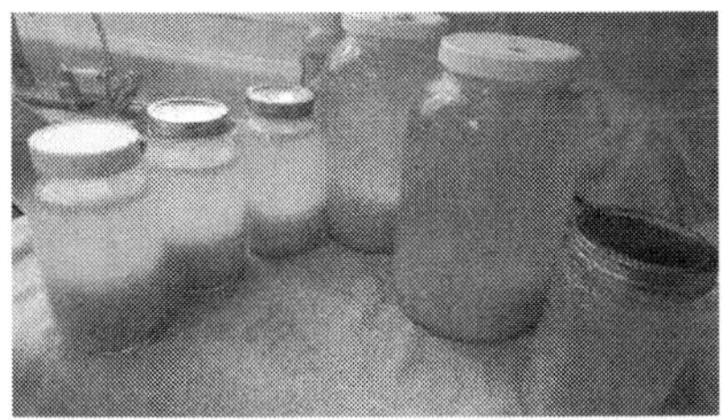

Making kraut juice is possibly the easiest and cheapest probiotic you can make at home. Kraut juice is gentle on the stomach, which makes it easy for digestion, and it is encouraged from at the earliest stages of GAPS. Kraut juice will ease constipation and help repopulate your good gut flora. Kraut juice should be used slowly and with great observation if you have great damage in the microbiome and you are on early stage GAPS; die-off from the kraut juice will manifest long before constipation relief is seen.

There are many ways to make kraut juice.

1. You can juice a head of cabbage and ferment it. This is done by putting a head of cabbage through a juicer and filling a Mason jar with the juiced liquid. For one quart of juiced cabbage add one tablespoon of whey, dripped from home-fermented yogurt, sour cream or kefir. Instead of whey, you can use salt or half salt and half whey. You can also use a culture starter packet. All three variations do the same thing. This recipe will yield one quart of kraut juice from one medium to large head of cabbage.
2. You can make sauerkraut and drain the juice off the top of the jar. This will yield about one cup of kraut juice from one medium to large head of cabbage.

You can make sauerkraut and drain the juice off the top of the jar. This will yield about one cup of kraut juice from one medium to large head of cabbage.

You can use the recipe below of chopping and salting cabbage, and then adding filtered water proportionately to the jar. This will yield about three gallons of kraut juice from one medium to large head of cabbage.

Clinically, we've experimented with all three as well as with commercially purchased Bubbies brand sauerkraut. All three produced the same die-off in eight "canaries in the coalmine." The Bubbies juice produced less die-off, showing a weaker probiotic content than the home brew.

Be sure to use an organic head of cabbage. As previously stated, kraut and kraut juice have a higher vitamin C content than the head of cabbage used to make the kraut and kraut juice. Vitamin C is a fantastic detoxifier, vital to GAPS people, so you will want a head of cabbage with the most vitamin C possible – organic.

Take a medium to large head of cabbage, and chop it up in the Vitamix by floating cubes of cabbage. Floating cubes of cabbage is done by filling the Vitamix up with water until it is 2/3 full, and then adding chopped cabbage and pulsing the machine for a few seconds. Then pour the mixture through a colander, leaving the finely chopped cabbage to use for kraut or kraut juice. The cabbage can also be cut up in a food processor or with a mandolin. None of these are really needed but are used for example purposes. A knife is really all that is needed. The smaller the pieces are, the faster they will ferment. Sprinkle six tablespoons of salt on top and stir thoroughly. Now you have a couple of choices: pound the kraut or ignore it, letting it sit. If the cabbage is chopped into tiny pieces as shown below, it can sit. If the cabbage is larger in size (for example, if it has been sliced thinly with a knife), it needs to be pounded or massaged to open up the cell walls.

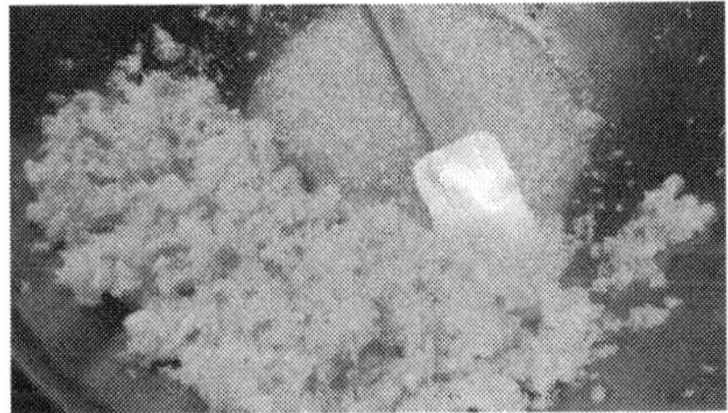

Let it sit anywhere from 20 minutes to overnight. The salt will do the work for you if your cabbage is shredded into small bits. What you are looking for is the extracted juices and opaque, limp cabbage. The salt is breaking down the cellular structure, releasing the juice of the cabbage.

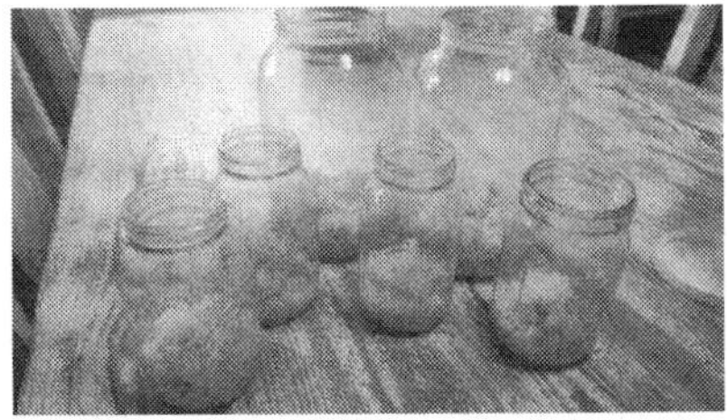

Fill your jars 1/3 of the way up with the cabbage and salt mixture. Fill the rest with filtered water.

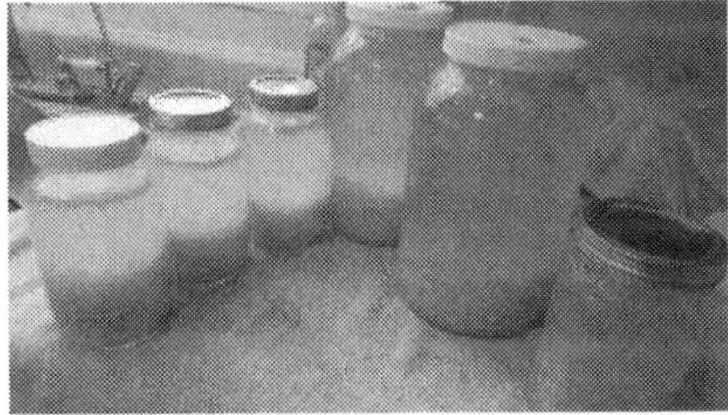

Put your lids on and let them to sit on the counter for nine to twelve days, preferably in a dark cool place. The amount of time for leaving kraut juice out as it brews depends on where you live —temperature is important. The other factors that make a huge difference in reference to mold growth are salt content and air. If air is accessible to your brew, it will mold faster. If leaving the brew out concerns you, do a shorter brew on the counter top, and then complete the brewing process in the refrigerator.

This will prevent mold growth.

There is no absolute rule on time for brewing, as these extra factors play an important role in the process. The variables of salt, air, sinking vs. floating vegetables, nutrients in the cabbage head, temperature, and sunlight all play a factor. You need to find what works best for you and your kitchen as well as what is tolerable to your body. "Canaries" with the deepest damage, those with histamine issues, have told us that the longer the ferment brews, the easier the product is tolerated. Those with the deepest gut damage to the microbiome need to allow their brew to sit for four months or longer for no histamine response.

Brewing jars like darker environments. Brewing under a towel in the corner of the countertop, near the air-conditioning vent, or in the basement is best. Sometimes the cabbage floats; sometimes it sinks — it really doesn't matter. If the kraut juice ferments for too long and white yeast forms on the top, kham yeast, just scoop it off and throw it away. The product is still good.

Refrigerate and enjoy.

There is great debate among home fermenters about mold, which can grow on top of the sauerkraut as it ferments. Mold happens due to oxidation, which is exposure to air. Some people say that if mold appears, the whole thing should be thrown out because the mold has tentacles that reach deep into the ferment.

This is, in no way, a unanimous thought amongst home fermenters.

Many people who have been fermenting for years, or traditional societies who have been fermenting for centuries, just scoop any mold off the top and eat the deeper sauerkraut.

The decision is yours.

Remember, it is the vegetable that sticks up and out of the brine that goes moldy from oxygen exposure.

People have been fermenting for centuries. Historically, this was the primary method of food preservation. Even Captain James Cook is famous for sauerkraut. Cook was an early explorer from the mid-1700s, a cartographer who supplied Britain, and the rest of the world, the first detailed map of the Pacific. He is famous for having a healthy crew when scurvy was very common among sailors. Cook sailed with barrels of sauerkraut on board, below deck. Of all the early explorers, Cook had the fewest number of deaths and the healthiest sailors.

When you consider the potential mold growth of sauerkraut on a ship rolling along the waves of the ocean, this method is not pristine. Considering their ability to keep the environment stable is encouraging to people making kraut for the first time. This is not a process of perfection.

Traditionally, Asian cultures bury their pots in the ground for fermentation. This is also not a pristine environment. The ground in one area is rocky; while in another, it is moist; in yet another, it is packed clay.

Yet, all environments are used, and the probiotic food product thrives.

Earlier generations stored their fermenting pots in the root cellar or in the corner of the room if they did not have land. Locations and environments of sauerkraut across the world, as well as vegetable preparation and varieties, have been countless. The conditions have been less than ideal as well as perfect.

Mold in the process of fermenting is not new.

Goitrogens And Fermented Food

Adverse side effects like malaise, weight gain, and exhaustion are being blamed on specific raw goitrogenic vegetables like cabbage, Brussel sprouts, broccoli, cauliflower, mustard greens, kale, turnips, and collards.

The *New England Journal of Medicine* reported a case in which an 88-year-old Chinese woman was trying to control her diabetes through eating bok choy, a Chinese cabbage. This goitrogenic vegetable is healthy, but for her, it became deadly.[ccxxix]

After she ate three to four heads a day, it damaged her thyroid to the point of crisis. After several months of her "healthy habit," she was so lethargic that she could not walk. Her throat began to close on her, and soon she could not swallow. After three days of extreme lethargy and an inability to swallow, she was taken to the emergency room.[ccxxx]

Her thyroid was not palpable, which means that it could not be felt to the touch; it was not engorged or filled with life.[ccxxxi]

She was suffering because vegetables from the brassica family were not well-tolerated by her body.[ccxxxii] Three to four heads of cabbage a day, for this woman, was clearly overdoing a good thing.

The *NEJM* reported that she experienced "respiratory failure and [was] admitted to the intensive care unit with a diagnosis of severe hypothyroidism with myxedema coma. She was treated with intravenous methylprednisolone and levothyroxine (thyroid medicines) and was eventually discharged."[ccxxxiii]

Brassica family vegetables contain compounds that are termed goitrogens because they inhibit the thyroid gland uptake of iodine.

In 1920, *The New Zealand Medical Journal* reported the deaths of two teenage girls and one teenage boy as the result of exophthalmic goiter, a result of thyroid deficiency.[ccxxxiv]

The *NZMJ* reported, "In 1928, Chesney and colleagues at Johns Hopkins found they could produce goiters in rabbits by feeding them a cabbage diet. This was the forerunner of medical treatment for thyrotoxicosis. Cabbage contained a positive goitrogenic substance, as opposed to the negative goitrogenic effect of iodine deficiency."[ccxxxv]

However, Dr. Barbara A. Hummel, a family medicine doctor at *Healthtap* says, "There are no food[s] that reverse hyperthyroidism or make it worse." Dr. Ed Friedlander agreed with her statement, as did Dr. Pamela Pappas and Dr. Alan Ali.[ccxxxvi]

The term goitrogen means goiter producer. A goiter is a growth on the thyroid gland.

Goitrogenic foods are known as being very beneficial for breast health; yet large amounts of uncooked goitrogens can suppress the thyroid by causing inflammation.

Cooking and fermenting goitrogens removes the problematic oxalic acid. This means that the elderly woman and three teenagers would have not had a thyroid issue if the cabbage had been made into sauerkraut.

A complete list of goitrogenic foods is as follows: kale, cabbage, collard greens, mustard greens, canola, kohlrabi, broccoli, Brussels sprouts, bok choy, rutabaga, turnip, cauliflower, radishes, millet, cassava, soy flour, soybean oil, soy lecithin, soy, strawberries, pears, peaches, and rapeseed.

However, avocado, coconut, caffeine, and saturated fat have also been shown to stimulate the thyroid.

Dr. Andrew Weil says, "Other foods that contain these chemicals include corn, sweet potatoes, lima beans, turnips, peanuts, cassava (yucca), canola oil and soybeans."[ccxxxvii]

Fortunately, the goitrogens in these foods are inactivated by cooking, even by light steaming, so there is no need to forgo on the valuable antioxidant and cancer-protective effects of cruciferous vegetables.

Cooking and fermenting changes the vegetable into a more digestible state.

The effects from vegetables that are goitrogens are negatively amplified if they are non-organic.

Juicing goitrogens brings a major concern of goitrogenic side effects when the vegetables are ingested in massive numbers, such as in the previously discussed case.

A better plan for juicing, it appears, would be juicing for variety: using cucumber or celery, which contain high quantities of potassium, with a low sugar hit like apples, carrots, and pineapple. To keep your health at an optimum level, choose non-goitrogenic vegetables for juicing, and be sure to eat all vegetables in organic form.

Juicing vegetables and drinking the brine from fermented vegetables share a common trait: they both go directly to the bloodstream. When vegetables are juiced, they lose their nutritional value as the time from juicing is extended. Generally, vegetables are healthiest directly after juicing and should be consumed within 20 minutes of juicing.

Only carrot juice is the exception to this rule. Carrot juice lasts up to two days in the refrigerator, even for those on the very strict Gerson Protocol.

However, fermented vegetable brine gets better over time. Fermentation of the vegetable opens up the cell walls and releases more nutrition into the brine. These brines are often timeless and mellow in flavor the longer they sit.

Both the freshly pressed juices and the fermented vegetable brine of these goitrogenic vegetables are delicious, but one of them can negatively impact a goiter, while the other carries probiotic strains and lasts for years.

Kombucha

The Central Laboratory for Analysis at the University of Science, Vietnam National University (VNU) ran a study on kombucha. They were trying to determine whether or not it was more effective to use added beneficial probiotic strains to the ferment. This has been a controversial topic for centuries.

"[Kombucha] is considered a health drink in many countries because it is a rich source of vitamins and may have other health benefits. It has previously been reported that adding lactic acid bacteria (*Lactobacillus*) strains to kombucha can enhance its biological functions, but in that study only lactic acid bacteria isolated from kefir grains were tested," says *Springer Plus*.[ccxxxviii]

The three main biological functions of kombucha are cited by the publication as glucuronic acid production, antibacterial activity, and antioxidant ability.[ccxxxix]

Glucuronic acid is non-toxic, organic acid that is the oxidation product of glucose. Glucuronic acid's main function is to attach to toxins and escort them out of the body.

The VNU study desired to show *Lactobacillus casei* and *Lactobacillus plantarum* from kefir and pickled cabbage to see if it would enhance kombucha's bioactivity. The kefir, pickled cabbage, and kombucha were obtained from a market in Ho Chi Minh City, Vietnam.[ccxl]

The kefir in the study was made from defatted homogeneous milk.[ccxli]

The study showed that the antibacterial and antioxidant activities of the kombucha were improved with the introduction of the *Lactobacillus casei* and *Lactobacillus plantarum*.

They found that, "on the fifth day of fermentation, the combination of strain lac5 and the [kombucha] layer produced 39.6% more GlcUA (glucuronic acid) than the original culture."[ccxlii]

This means that the kombucha produced more glucuronic acid, enabling the body to eliminate more toxins and to have higher antibacterial and antioxidant ability.

The International Journal of Cell Biology says that glucuronic acid is known to be effective against cancer.[ccxliii]

In another study, kombucha was tested to determine its wound healing effects. It was tested on mice against an antibacterial ointment, Nitrofurazone, which is a wound and hoof care ointment used for bacterial infections of wounds, burns, and cutaneous ulcers. *Diagnostic Pathology* reported the study.[ccxliv]

Federal law restricts against the use of Nitrofurazone, prohibiting the use of this product in food-producing animals. It stands to reason that a natural product that accomplishes the same results would be optimal to use, since food-producing animals tend to get wounds, burns, and cutaneous ulcers.[ccxlv]

They said, "The clinical findings indicated that the [k]ombucha fungus resulted in precipitating [more] healing than Nitrofurazone. [...] Several wound biopsies were taken on 4, 8, 12, 16 and 20th days. [*sic*]"[ccxlvi]

They further reported, "Additionally, the histopathological results demonstrated that there was inflammation in Nitrofurazone group through [the] twelfth day[;] somehow the epithelium was formed and abundant vessels were visible. Although on [the] 16th day and the previous days[,] the healing condition of [the k]ombucha fungus was considered as minimal rate, revealing it is similar to Nitrofurazone group on [the] 20th day."[ccxlvii]

What they are saying is that a medicinal cream and kombucha were both used topically to heal wounds on animals. The medicinal cream and kombucha performed with similar healing outcomes, with kombucha favored. The medicinal cream showed greater inflammation than the kombucha, even up to the twelfth day.[ccxlviii]

The Serbian publication *Acta Periodica Technologica* says, "Acetic acid, Kombucha samples and heat denaturated [kombucha] showed significant antimicrobial activity against bacteria. However, there was no activity against yeasts and molds. Kombucha showed higher antioxidant activity than tea."[ccxlix]

Some studies show that kombucha is high in B vitamins; however, the B vitamin group is not the only key player.

Springer Plus published a study saying, "The bacterial component of [k]ombucha cultures [...] is known to comprise several species, including acetic acid bacteria." It also claims that "the antioxidant properties of [k]ombucha may be high because vitamin C, vitamin B and DSL [(D-saccharic acid 1,4 lactone)] are synthesized during fermentation."[ccl]

In addition to the drink itself being so high in B vitamins, the combination of other benefits with the B vitamins boosts the function of the body, acting much like B vitamins – only better and more complete. This happens due to the vitamin B, high antioxidant factor, vitamin C, and D-saccharic acid 1, 4 lactone (DSL) working so well in the body that it causes multiple subsequent health benefits.[ccli]

If kombucha has high vitamin B levels, high antioxidant factors, vitamin C, and D-saccharic acids, it is classified in the same category as vitamin supplements.

Free Radical Research reported a study using DSL, like the one found in kombucha, in diabetic induced rats. It found that a dose of 80 mg of kombucha per kg of body weight restored alterations in diabetic rats. It led to proper cell death, mitochondrial repair, protection of the spleen, and correction of hyperglycemia. It was determined that this aspect of the diet could lessen diabetes associated spleen dysfunction.[cclii]

Medline Plus says, "There is some concern that kombucha tea might decrease niacin absorption."[ccliii] This needs to be studied more because niacin deficiencies present as fears, anxiety, depression, bipolar behavior, and schizophrenia. Those taking kombucha do not show these signs; in fact, they show the opposite.

Niacin is vitamin B3.

The Mayo Clinic says that kombucha "contains vinegar, B vitamins and a number of other chemical compounds."[ccliv]

They go on to say, "At the same time, several cases of harm have been reported. Therefore, the prudent approach is to avoid kombucha tea until more definitive information is available."[cclv]

This poses many questions. Why do we need to avoid a product, being "prudent" as they say, until further studies are performed, when traditional cultures have been fermenting tea into kombucha for centuries without incident?

The cases that caused harm were reported by the CDC. Studying their findings may prevent us from throwing the proverbial baby out with the bathwater.[cclvi]

It is important to note that the two cases discussed and reported as the concern for kombucha awareness and studies are of women who knew each other. These two women lived in the same town and shared the same SCOBY with each other.[cclvii] A SCOBY is a Symbiotic Colony of Bacterial Yeasts, the starter for brewing kombucha. It can also be called a starter, a mother, a pancake or a mushroom.

Once we know more about a situation, we can do better.

Case one:

> A 59-year-old woman was taken to the emergency room after she was found unconscious. Arterial blood samples showed severe metabolic acidosis with a pH of 6.9 (normal levels are 7.37-7.43) and an elevated lactic acid level of 9.85mM (normal is 0.67mM-2.47mM). She had been taking medication for hypertension, anemia, and renal insufficiency.[cclviii]
>
> In the hospital, she showed symptoms of disseminated intravascular coagulopathy, which presents with blood clots and bleeding. She experienced cardiac arrest and was resuscitated; however, her health continued to decline. She died two days after being admitted to the hospital.[cclix]
>
> The autopsy showed peritonitis, leakage or hole in the intestinal tract, which can be caused by many reasons such as a burst appendix.[cclx]
>
> There was fecal contamination in the peritoneal cavity, although a perforation of the intestinal tract could not be found. Peritonitis, which is usually life threatening, consists of inflammation of the membrane lining the abdominal wall as well as the membrane covering the abdominal organs. Most often peritonitis is infectious and life-threatening. Protocol consists of using antibiotics, along with surgery or drainage.[cclxi]
>
> The woman was taking 4 ounces of kombucha daily for two months prior to her death.[cclxii]
>
> Those studying her case thought kombucha to be a major player in her death. No studies are reported of studying her medicines or other heath conditions.[cclxiii]

Case two:

Seven days after the first woman passed away, another woman, 48 years of age, went to the same emergency room, by ambulance, with shortness of breath. Tests showed extensive fluid in the lungs.

Blood tests showed elevated pH levels. She suffered cardiac arrest, was resuscitated, improved, and was discharged three days after admission.[cclxiv]

No drugs, prescription or otherwise, were found in her system. No cause of the cardiac event was found. She had been drinking kombucha for two months. Immediately prior to her symptoms, she had increased her consumption of kombucha from four ounces a day to 12 ounces a day. She had also just changed her brew time from seven days to fourteen days.[cclxv]

Authorities began to investigate and found that 115 people in the town were brewing and drinking kombucha from the same starter SCOBY, which had been purchased by one individual from a commercial supplier and shared among friends and family members in the town. The average drinker in the town was 57.1 years old. No other illnesses were reported by any other kombucha drinkers. Hospital records showed no other related cases of lactic acidosis.[cclxvi]

The FDA (Federal Drug Association) tested the tea and SCOBY from both the case one patient and the case two patient, as well as from the other kombucha brewers and drinkers in the town.[cclxvii]

In the samples, scientists found several yeasts and bacteria. *Sacchromyces cerevisiae* was found.[cclxviii] *S. cerevisiae* is a sugar fungus, meaning that it feeds on glucose. It eats sugar and off-gasses carbon dioxide and ethanol. It is commonly known as brewer's, baker's yeast, or brewer's yeast; it is not nutritional yeast but the two are often confused for being the same thing. It is found naturally in wine and beer fermentation.

Nutrients says, "*Saccharomyces cerevisiae*, which according to EFSA (The European Food Safety Authority) has a QPS (Qualified Presumption of Safety) status, is the most common yeast used in food fermentation."[cclxix]

They go on to say, "The electrophoretic karyotypes of the *S. boulardii* strains appeared quite uniform and although very typical of *S. cerevisiae*, they formed a cluster separate from other strains within this species. The results of the study strongly indicated a close relatedness of *S. boulardii* to *S. cerevisiae* and thereby support the recognition of *S. boulardii* as a member of *S. cerevisiae* and not as a separate species. Strains of *S. boulardii* should be seen as a separate cluster within the *S. cerevisiae* species."[cclxx] *Sacchromyces boulardii* is known to keep pathogenic yeasts under control. However, it is not recommended as an isolated strain; it works best with supporting nutrients and beneficial strains. In kombucha, it has these supporting strains naturally.

Therapeutic Advances in Gastroenterology says, "Several clinical trials and experimental studies strongly suggest a place for *Saccharomyces boulardii* as a biotherapeutic agent for the prevention and treatment of several gastrointestinal diseases. *S. boulardii* mediates responses resembling the protective effects of the normal healthy gut flora. The multiple mechanisms of action of *S. boulardii* and its properties may explain its efficacy and beneficial effects in acute and chronic gastrointestinal diseases that have been confirmed by clinical trials."[cclxxi]

Scientists also found *Candida valida* in the kombucha samples tested. They did not find any toxin-producing organisms or pathogens in any of the samples tested. *Candida valida* is another beneficial form of Candida, supportive of the system.

This is proven time and time again when people who are sensitive to yeast issues show no disturbance with long-brewed kombucha. It is also proven when children with eczema, or other yeasts, drink kombucha. They are hypersensitive to yeasts and molds, yet they get better on kombucha. It is wise to note that the ladies in the study were drinking 4 ounces of kombucha or an increased number of 12 ounces of kombucha. Many of the hypersensitive children are drinking several quarts a day. Some are drinking four quarts a day. This would equal 64 ounces or 128 ounces.

Kombucha contains butyric acid, which assists in cellular membrane health. The glucuronic acid found in kombucha is known to strengthen the walls of the intestinal tract.[cclxxii]

"The microbial community of [k]ombucha tea consists of bacteria and yeast which thrive in two mutually non-exclusive compartments: the soup or the beverage and the biofilm floating on it," says *Internal Journal of Food Microbiology*.[cclxxiii]

The journal tested the tea beverage at different times up to 21 days of fermentation.[cclxxiv]

They found that "the yeast community of the biofilm did not show much variation over time and was dominated by *Candida sp.* (73.5-83%). The soup however, showed a significant shift in dominance from *Candida sp.* to *Lachancea sp.* on the 7th day of fermentation. This is the first report showing Candida as the most dominating yeast genus during [k]ombucha fermentation. Komagateibacter was identified as the single largest bacterial genus present in both the biofilm and the soup (~50%)."[cclxxv] As we already know, there are good bacteria and bad bacteria, as well as good yeasts and pathogenic yeasts.

This includes good Candida and bad Candida. The Candida in kombucha is classified as beneficial.

Bacteria are decomposers, breaking down matter. In the forest, bacteria break down decaying leaves and wood. This feeds the soil.

"The bacterial diversity was higher in the soup than in the biofilm with a peak on the seventh day of fermentation. The biochemical properties changed with the progression of the fermentation, i.e., beneficial properties of the beverage such as the radical scavenging ability increased significantly with a maximum increase at day 7," they reported.[cclxxvi]

The American Society for Microbiology, Genome Announcements tested booch (kombucha's nickname) and found that "*Komagataeibacter intermedius* AF2, previously known as *Gluconacetobacter intermedius*, is a Gramnegative rod isolated from kombucha tea."[cclxxvii]

The tea was plated, incubated aerobically, and analyzed. They discovered that *Komagataeibacter intermedius* AF2 produced 1.41 g/L of cellulose and found "gene content similar to related species: *K. rhaeticus* (3,460 genes), *K. xylinus* (3,195), *K. hansenii* (3,308), *K. medellinensis* (3,195), *K. europaeus* 5P3 (3,586), *K. oboediens* 174Bp2 (3,601), and *G. diazotrophicus* (3,864)."[cclxxviii]

Gluconacetobacter produces cellulose, a chain of linked sugar molecules. Cellulose, in its natural form, is in vegetables. It holds the cell walls together, giving the plant strength.

Kombucha is a known *Acetobacteraceae* family habitat. *Molekuliarnaia Biologiia* says, "Acetobacteraceae are often hard to culture in laboratory conditions and they also maintain very low abundances in their natural habitats. Thus identification of the organisms in such environments is greatly dependent on modern tools of molecular biology which require a thorough knowledge of specific conserved gene sequences that may act as primers and or probes." [*sic*][cclxxix]

Food Chemistry reported a study testing 10 different types of tea used to ferment kombucha. They found that "an enhancement of the antioxidant and starch hydrolase inhibitory potential of the herbal teas was observed by adding the tea fungus."[cclxxx]

This means that the medicinal aspects of herbal teas were enhanced when fermented into booch.

Different herbal teas have different medicinal properties. Stinging nettles herbal tea is known for reducing and subsequently draining inflamed lymph nodes. Peppermint herbal tea is known as a digestive aid. Licorice root is known to support the adrenals. Chamomile is known for having sedative effects, calming a person down. Green tea is a known antioxidant. Rooibos tea is known for assisting the body in making glutathione. Wild mint is known for aiding in digestion. Ginger tea is a prokinetic, meaning that it reactivates the functions of the digestive tract that may have been negatively impacted from pathogenic flora. It has been shown to support activation of the migrating motor complex, a digestive function in the small intestine that pushes and sweeps pathogens down into the large intestine. It also demonstrates the ability to strengthen the ileocecal valve, which separates pathogenic flora from the small intestine and the large intestine.

If these medicinal teas are amplified in their medicinal properties, assisting people with damaged microbiomes, as shown in this study, their support would be remarkable.

This study, however, was retracted, citing "article withdrawal."

Article withdrawal happens for "potential error content or possible infringements of professional ethical codes such as multiple submission, bogus claims of authorship, plagiarism, fraudulent use of data or the like."[cclxxxi]

The article showed "the enhancement of antioxidant and starch hydrolase inhibitory properties."[cclxxxii]

The *Journal of Food Science and Technology* reported a study on kombucha, which they also call bio-tea. In the study, rats with myocardial damage were tested. They stated, "Traditional claims about kombucha report beneficial effects such as antibiotic properties, gastric regulation, relief from joint rheumatism and positive influence on the cholesterol level, arteriosclerosis, diabetes, and aging problems."[cclxxxiii]

They found that "bio-tea showed a higher preventive effect against myocardial infarction when compared to tea, as was observed by the significant reduction in heart weight, and blood glucose and increase in plasma albumin levels. Bio-tea significantly decreased cholesterol, triglycerides, LDL and VLDL while simultaneously increasing the levels of HDL. Similarly, a decrease in leakage of cardiac markers from the myocardium was also observed."[cclxxxiv]

One study published in *Pharmaceutical Biology* showed the effects on rats fed a cholesterol-rich diet for 16 weeks as compared with the effects of the addition of kombucha to a cholesterol-rich diet. They found that "KT [kombucha tea] induced a 55% decrease of TBARS level in liver and 44% in kidney, compared with those of rats fed a cholesterol-rich diet alone. Moreover, CAT and SOD activities were reduced by 29 and 33%, respectively, in liver and 31 and 35%, respectively, in kidney, after oral administration of KT."[cclxxxv] TBARS develop as fats and are processed in the liver, resulting in cell damage. The oxidative stress of this process leads to disease.[cclxxxvi] They found that kombucha assists the body in processing the fats.[cclxxxvii] Therefore, some people who are very in tune with their body crave kombucha after they have eaten a fat laden meal. It helps process the lipids.

In layman's terms, this means that kombucha supported the liver and kidney function with a remarkable effect. Cell damage was less with kombucha support. Disease was less notable. The kombucha assisted in cutting and processing the extra fat from the meal, allowing the body to use it as nourishment.

The *International Journal of Food Microbiology* reported the study saying, "We further observed a significantly higher D-saccharic acid-1,4-lactone content and caffeine degradation property compared to previously described kombucha tea fermentations."[cclxxxviii]

Higher D-saccharic acid, 4-lactone levels in the body have been shown to support the spleen, reversing diabetes.[cclxxxix]

They concluded, "The findings revealed that KT administration induced attractive curative effects on hypercholesterolemi[a], particularly in terms of liver-kidney functions in rats."[ccxc]

This means that the beneficial aspects of kombucha support the spleen, acting as a retardant to diabetes.

These aspects in kombucha result from the processed caffeine in the brewing process.

This also means, if the articles above stand true, that the medicinal properties of herbal teas used in making kombucha tea should be combined with caffeinated teas. This includes black tea, which is traditionally used in making kombucha.

Food and Agriculture Immunology published a study done on 18 mice fed kombucha, which showed that "images of stained tissue sections from all groups demonstrated that inflammation criteria and demyelination in mice treated by [k]ombucha tea were significantly less than control mice."[ccxci]

This means that the mice treated with kombucha had better nerve signaling activity.

They further added, "Staining of brains [*sic*] sections showed that kombucha tea therapy could suppress the progression of inflammation significantly."[ccxcii]

The *Journal of Microbiology and Biotechnology* printed a study on kombucha finding booch has "the potential to revert the CCl4-induced hepatotoxicity. Antioxidant molecules produced during the fermentation period could be the reason for the efficient hepatoprotective and curative properties of KT against CCl4-induced hepatotoxicity."[ccxciii]

In layman's terms, this means that kombucha showed curative properties on liver damage.

The *Journal of Food Protection* says, "Kombucha has in vitro antimicrobial activity and enhances sleep and pain thresholds in rats."[ccxciv]

BioMed Central Complementary and Alternative Medicine reported a study on diabetic rats that lasted 31 days. According to the study, "the findings revealed that kombucha tea administration induced attractive curative effects on diabetic rats, particularly in terms of liver-kidney functions. Kombucha tea can, therefore, be considered as a potential strong candidate for future application as a functional supplement for the treatment and prevention of diabetes."[ccxcv]

Researchers in the study induced brain inflammation in the animals. Inflammation in the mice "was delayed in [k]ombucha tea-treated mice compared to control mice."[ccxcvi]

Compacting this down, these studies are showing that kombucha enhances antioxidants, assists the body in processing starches, assists in supporting blood sugar levels, assists the body in processing fats, assists against a heart attack, supports the liver and kidney function, supports the spleen to ward off diabetes, gives energy through proper transactions of B vitamins, topically assists in healing wounds, topically assists in healing burns, assists in the function of nerve connections, has many beneficial yeasts and bacteria, and reduces inflammation.

“Kombucha’s great, especially for women, particularly to detoxify from estrogens,” says Dr. Patrick Vickers.[ccxcvii] Vickers resides in Mexico where he runs the Northern Baja Gerson Center.

"The liver has five pathways that it detoxifies. One of those pathways is the glucoronodation pathway. That's actually very specific for estrogen detoxification,” says Dr. Vickers.[ccxcviii]

One natural food product that assists with this process is kombucha.

"If you look on a kombucha bottle in the store you'll see it has high amounts of glycosidase. That shuttles estrogens through the liver pathway for estrogen detoxification,"[ccxcix] Vickers says.

There are several reasons for estrogen to be in an overloaded state, including soy-based foods, plastics in our food preparation, BPAs from coffee cup lids and water bottles, as well as from other acidic or heated foods which come in contact with plastic, and illness. Getting this overflow out of the system taxes the body. If it cannot escape, the imbalance from the overflow creates other imbalances and can snowball downhill. Opening the detox pathways, specific to each person, assists the body with normal functions.

Dr. Vickers goes on to say, "In cases where hormones might be out of control – great supplement."[ccc]

Vickers works in alternative therapy through The Gerson Treatment. Kombucha, and other fermented vegetables, are not part of the Gerson plan. When referring to estrogen overflow and cancer, he does not recommend kombucha as part of the Gerson Protocol.

For others, it is highly beneficial.

Kombucha candy is a healthful treat that travels well and provides a tasty alternative to sweets.

When your kombucha makes the extra SCOBY and there's no one waiting in line for a starter, peel off the extra layer.

The thinner the SCOBY is, the more it will look like stained glass candy. The thicker the SCOBY is, the more it will respond like taffy. Cut the SCOBY with stainless steel scissors, and then lay them out on dehydrator trays. Drizzle a thin line of local honey and salt on the SCOBY strips, and dehydrate on 115 degrees overnight or until your desired firmness. SCOBY strips can also be marinated in honey and sprinkled with salt prior to dehydrating.

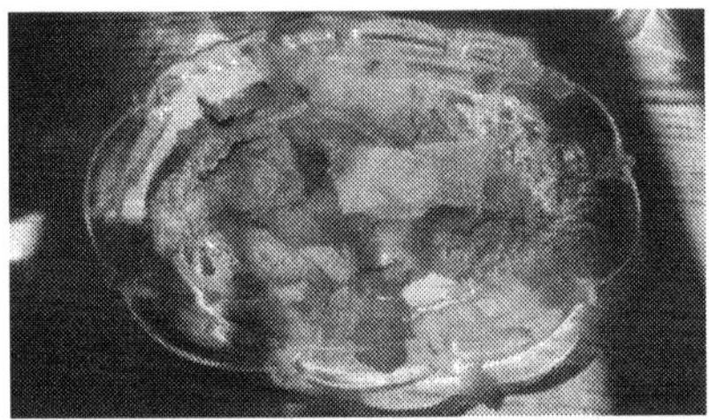

These treats travel well for hikes or air travel and provide a boost from the many beneficial aspects of the kombucha SCOBY.

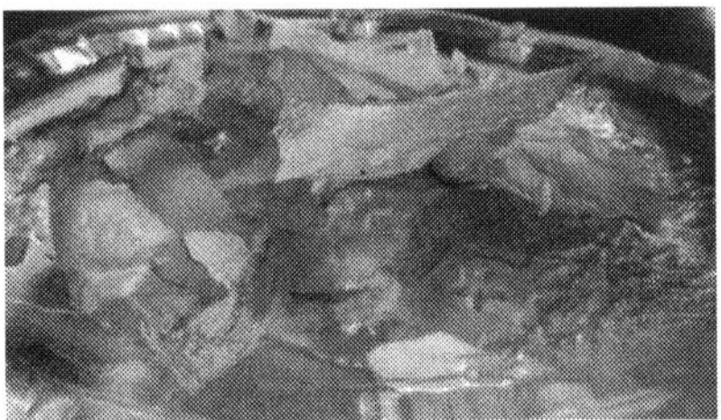

Gargling with kombucha is a deeper method of cleansing the membranes from potential pathogens, parasites, and excess mucus. The method is simple: take a good-sized drink of (preferably) home brewed kombucha; tilt your head back and forcefully gargle until you are out of breath; tilt your head forward; inhale (be careful to not swallow or spit); gargle again until you are out of breath; lean forward and inhale again; gargle again; spit.

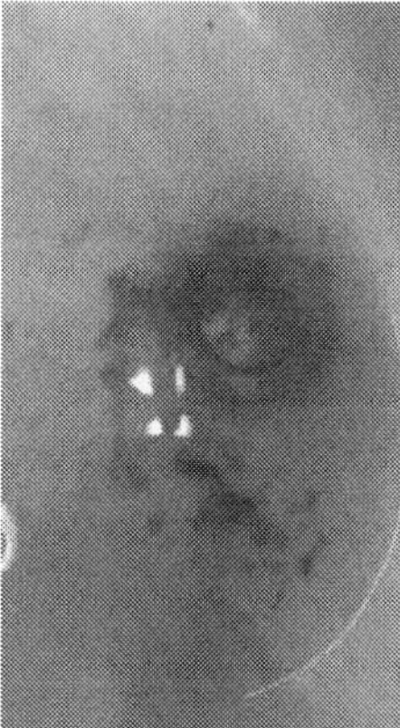

Some people believe the expelled contents are parasites and worms. It resembles mucus.

Following the same process with water leaves no result. This sample below was done with clear water immediately after the kombucha gargle.

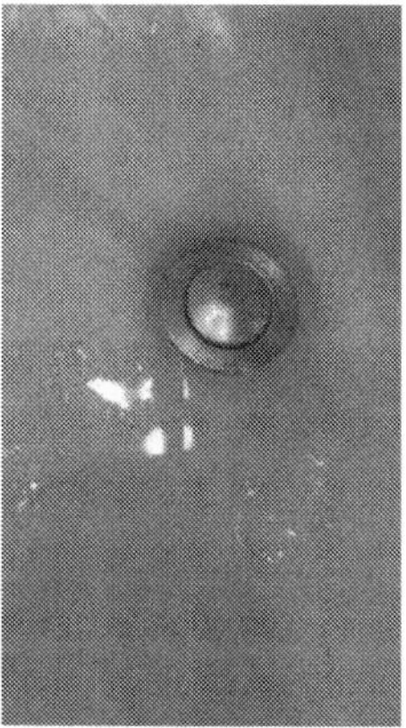

Immediately following the water gargle, this is another sample using the same pattern of gargle, inhale, gargle, inhale, gargle, spit with another dose of kombucha. The results again produce the mucous worm-like substances.

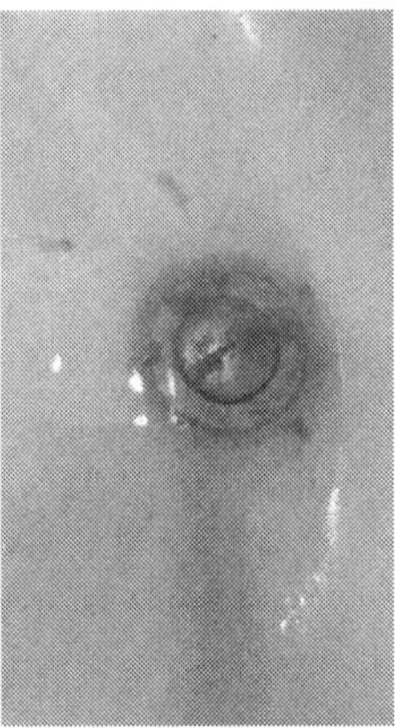

No studies have been done on this method; this is purely a trial and error method of potential cleansing.

Some believe it is a possible residue of the kombucha, as it resembles floating particles in the kombucha brew. However, when you put the kombucha in the mouth and let it sit, it doesn't have floaters. When you put kombucha in a glass and shake it, to simulate the same action, there are no floaters. If the kombucha were forming these floaters by separating, it would leave us to believe that the kombucha would separate with the shaking in the glass, also.

In recent years, a mommy blogger has tried to vilify kombucha due to the fluoride content of teas. Other bloggers were questioned as to why they continued to support the use of kombucha with the reports of fluoride existing in tea. Posts like these can bring great confusion to people trying to do their best with probiotic foods. As Codlivergate (concerns over fermented cod liver oil) divided the masses, the fluoride in kombucha scare caused people to stop making probiotic foods for their families.

It is important to remember that many foods (not just tea leaves) contain natural levels of fluoride. In addition, drinking a cup of tea uses one to two tea bags, whereas fermenting kombucha uses 8 to 12 teabags for a gallon. Those who are familiar with the function of halides in the body will tell you that fluoride, as well as chloride and bromide, cannot fill receptor cells when there are appropriate iodine levels present.

Many children, as well as immunocompromised teenagers, adults, and elderly, drink kombucha, with some reporting over 4 quarts a day. Toddlers drink kombucha as an exchange for juice as well.

No high levels of fluoride, or fluorosis, including mottling of teeth or calcification of ligaments, have emerged. Instead, these individuals show positive results.

The body processes minerals and nutrition in its own way. When we analyze foods in the lab, it is a simulation. When we break down the content of foods in a lab, the methods and products that are used to break down the foods and decipher their content are different from how our bodies process these foods.

People have been drinking tea for centuries.

Some southerners drink sweet tea by the gallon each day in the summertime.

Although tea shows fluoride levels in the lab, reports of high levels of fluoride or fluorosis have not been reported from drinking tea or kombucha, even though the quantity consumed through recorded history has been in copious amounts.

Dentists and dental hygienists do, however, report teeth straining from drinking tea. They do not show the same for kombucha consumption.

Kombucha SCOBY, Moldy or Good?

Making kombucha for the first time is a bit scary. When the SCOBY begins to grow, sometimes it is hard to determine the difference between a moldy SCOBY and the standard SCOBY growing process. This collage of pictures, listed below, can help you decide.

There is a lot of forgiveness in making kombucha. In fact, it is hard to have the SCOBY go moldy; it is a very rare occurrence. Reports show one moldy SCOBY out of every 50,000 gallons brewed.

Mold grows on kombucha, on average, less than one percent of the time.

If the SCOBY does go moldy, it should be discarded, along with all the kombucha it brewed. If you are in doubt and the booch looks like it is growing mold, the easiest thing to do is wait.

When the new SCOBY (also known as mother, starter, mushroom, culture, or pancake) is forming, it often looks like mold is growing. If there is concern of mold, give it a few days to rest, and see if the mold has advanced into green, black, or white mold. True mold on a SCOBY is usually purple in color.

Most likely, it is simply the SCOBY growing properly.

As the booch brews, it grows another SCOBY, which can have a deceptive appearance, looking like mold.

Waiting will answer the question.

If, in fact, there is mold, it will remain on the surface of the SCOBY, looking like a green- or purple- hued, bumpy mold. The color of mold growing on a SCOBY is remarkably vibrant. A new SCOBY will still form over top of problematic mold, but it will take well over a month for the mold to be covered over with the new SCOBY.

A normal SCOBY will form in roughly seven days of brewing. If there appears to be mold, and it truly is mold, the newly formed SCOBY cannot form on top in the seven days' time.

If you think the SCOBY is growing mold, wait a couple of days and see if it is just the new SCOBY growing. Like most things, the first brew is the hardest. Once you get past the learning curve, you will wonder why you waited so long.

These pictures are all healthy SCOBYs.

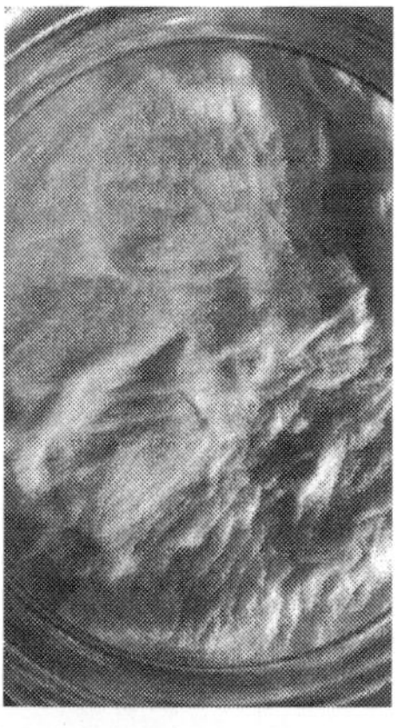

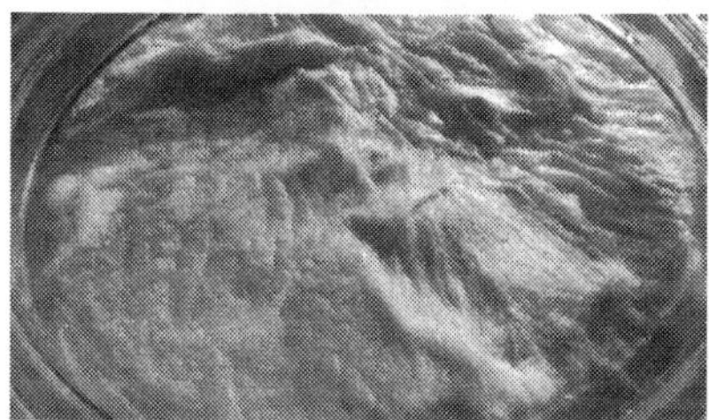

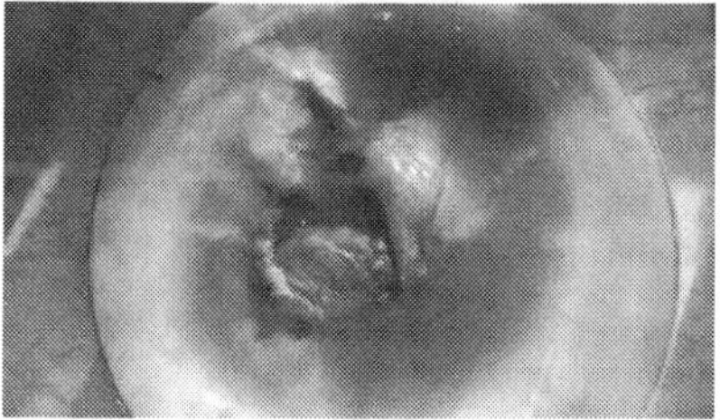

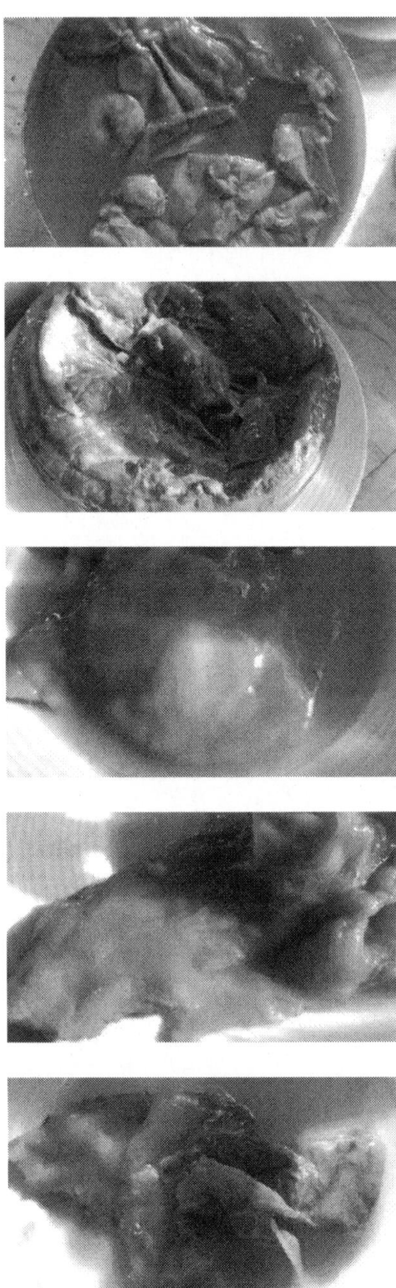

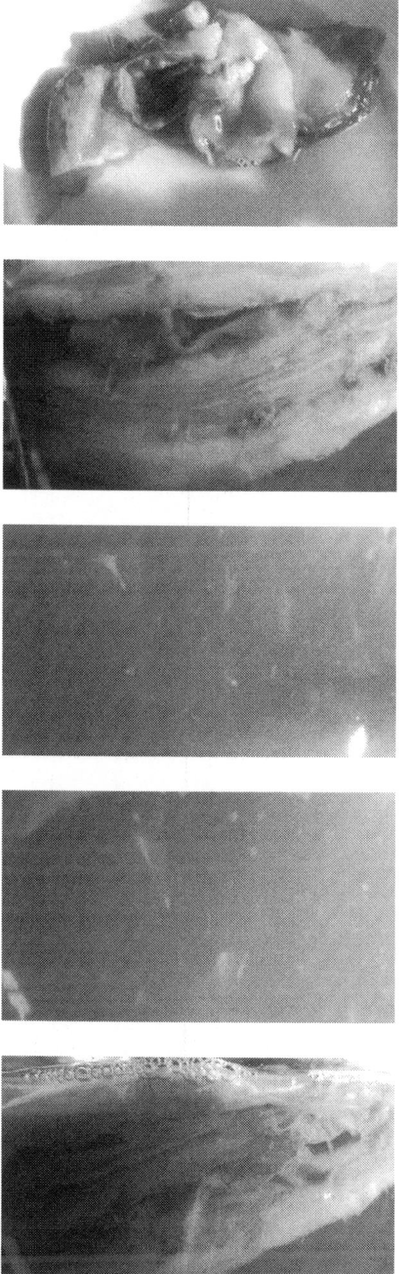

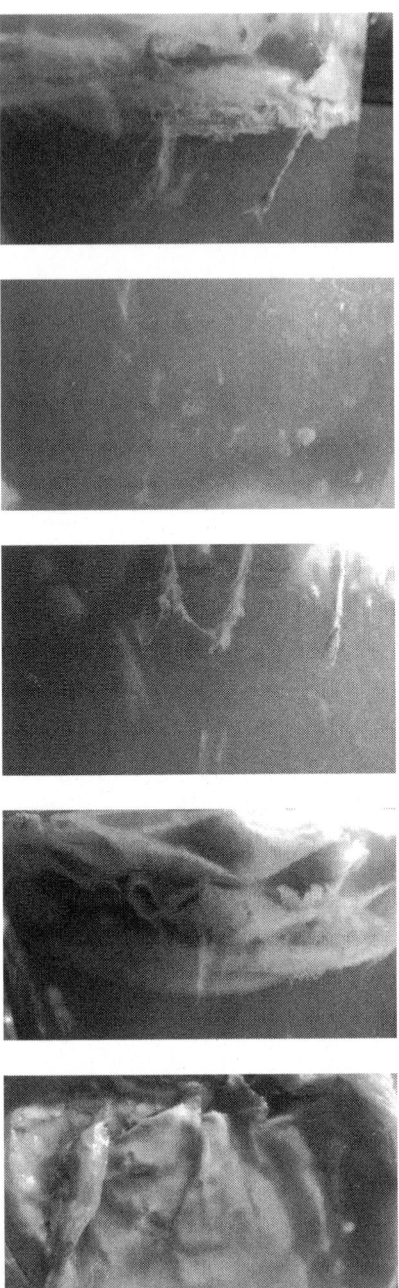

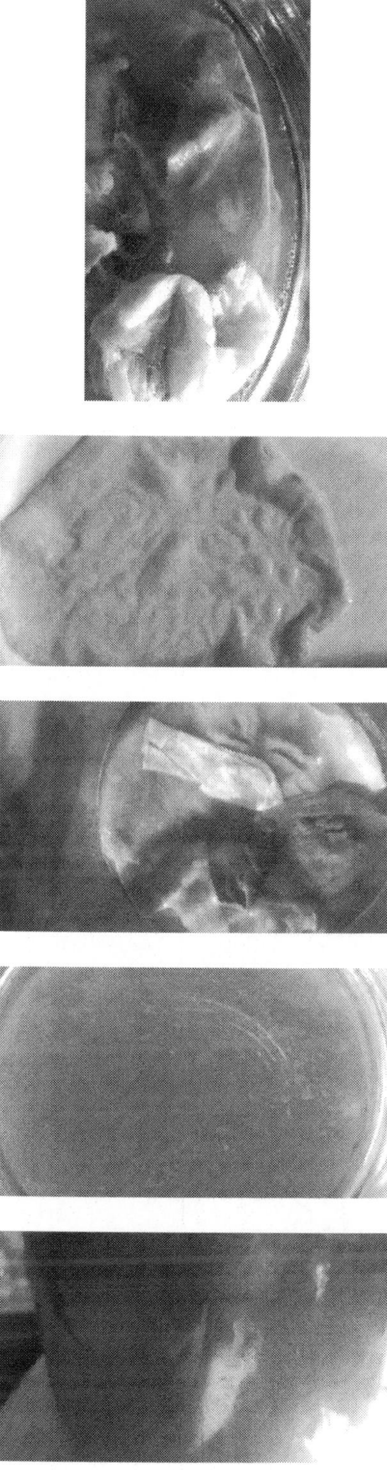

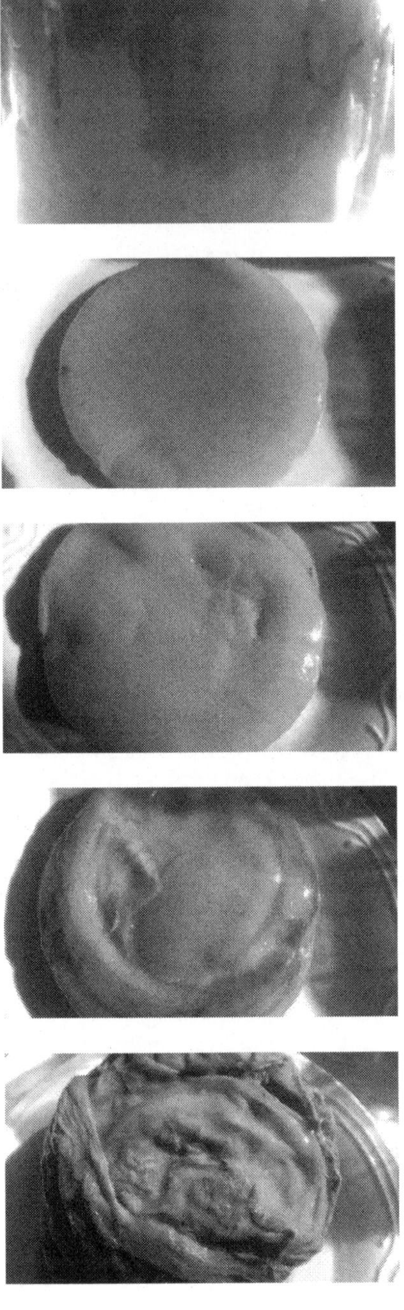

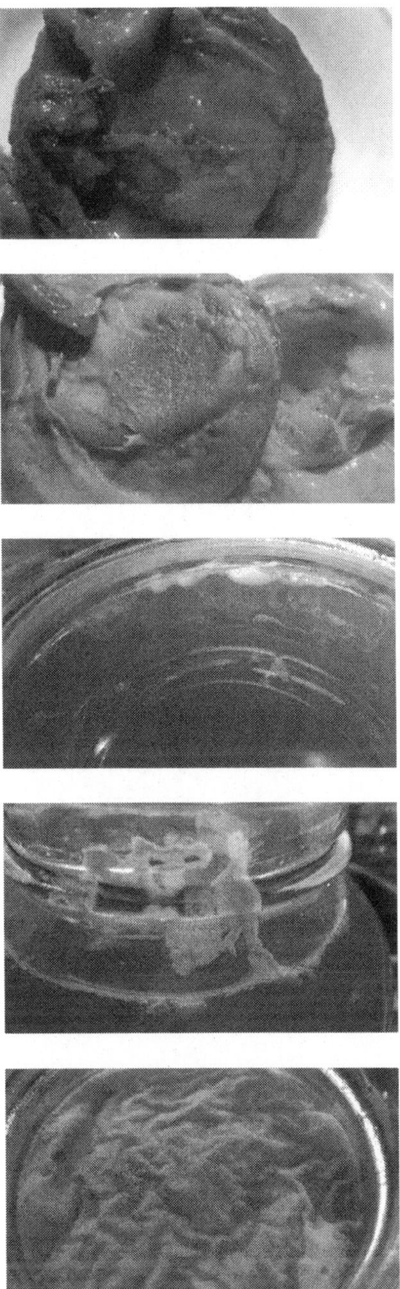

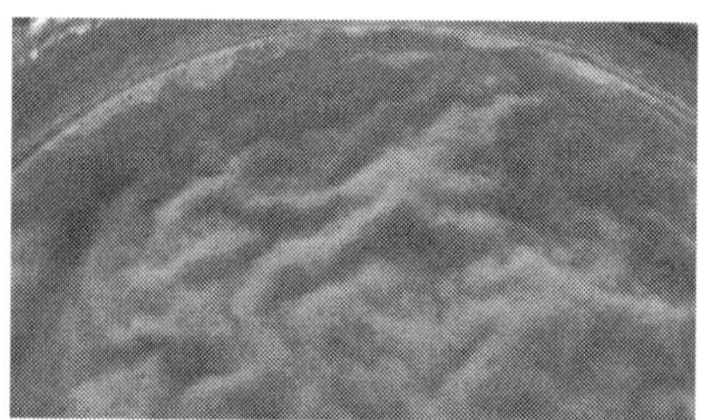

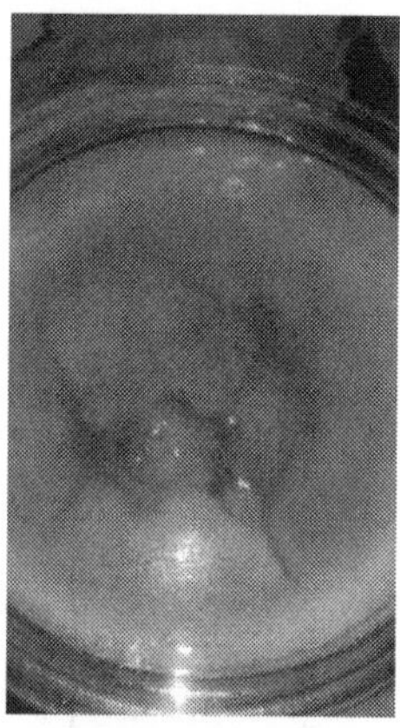

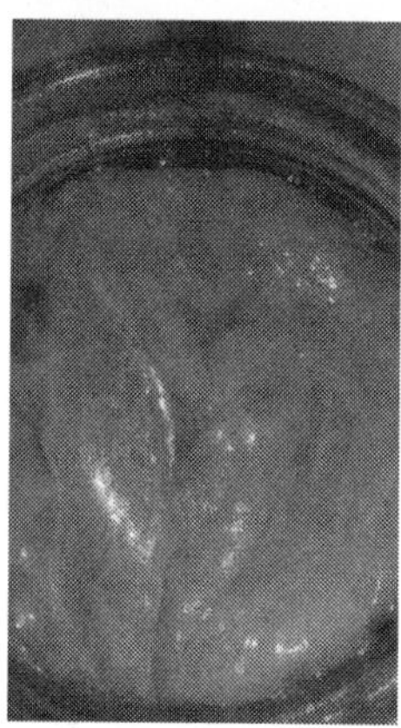

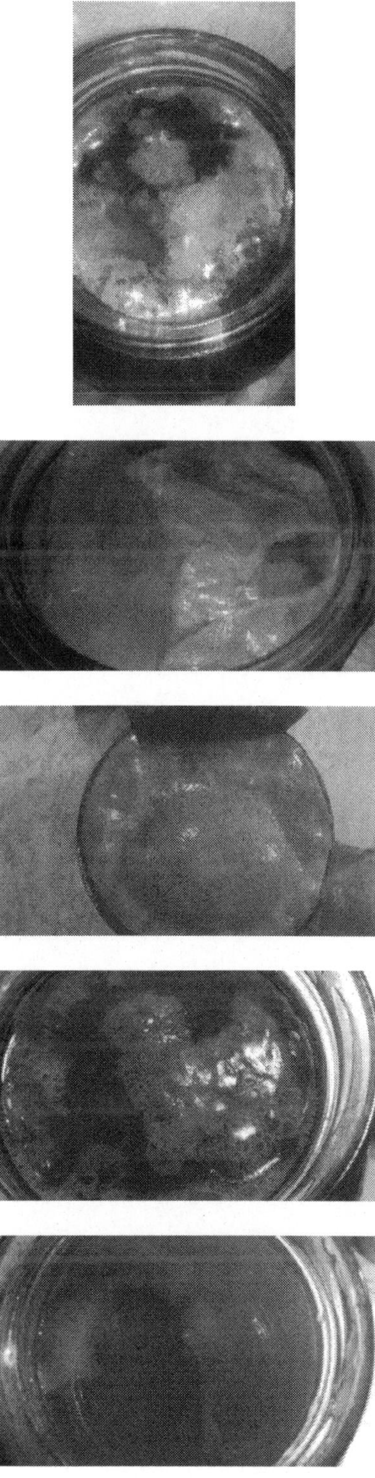

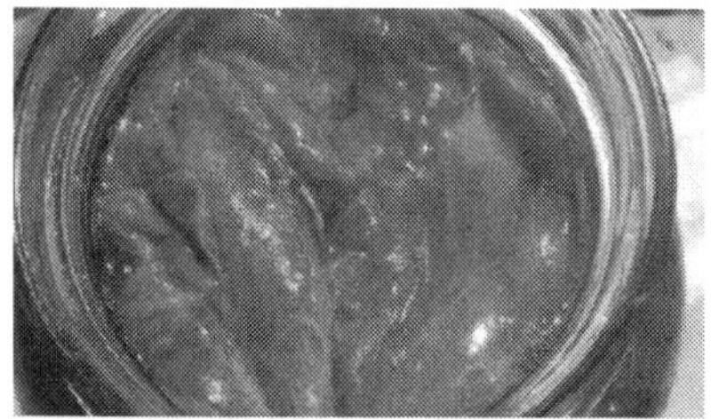

This is what a moldy SCOBY looks like. Take note of the purple hue, which is vibrant, not subdued, in color.

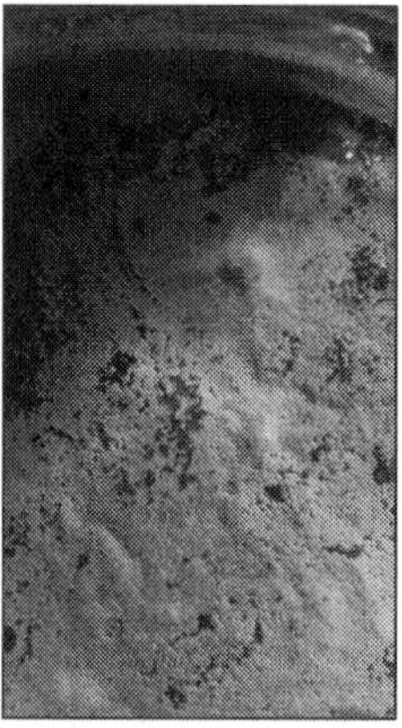

Again, if it is moldy, the new growth on top of the mold takes about a month and a half to two months to grow the new mushroom over the mold layer. A healthy SCOBY grows in roughly one week.

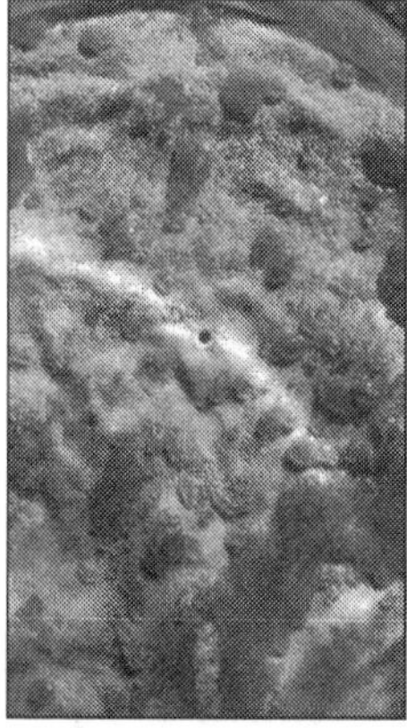

As the new mushroom begins to grow on top of the mold, it looks like little gel bubbles.

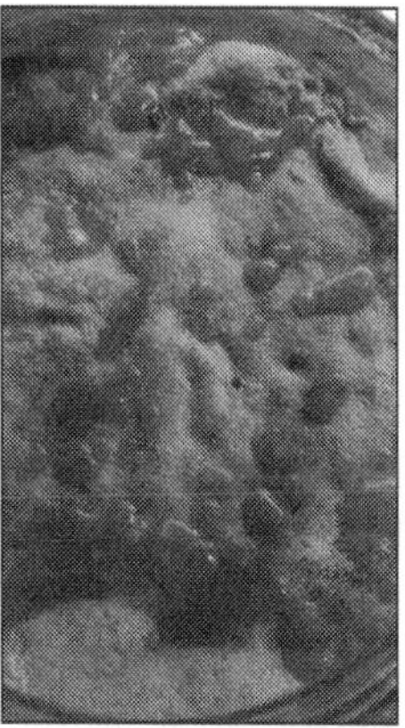

After roughly a week, the small bubbles are slightly bigger and connect. Again, a normal mushroom is complete in one week.

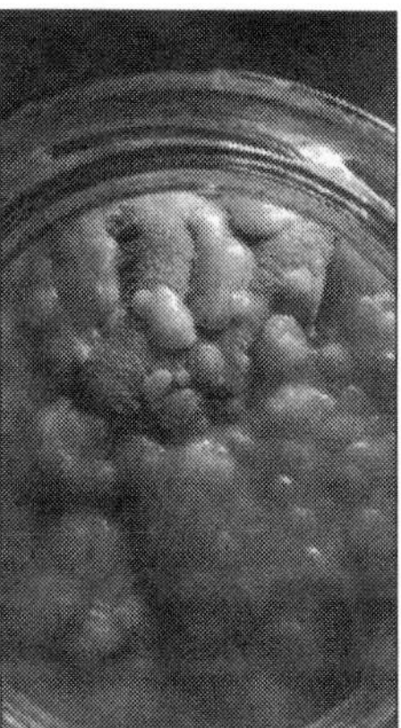

After well over a month, the mushroom is almost fully formed on top of the mold. This should not be eaten. The whole vessel of tea as well as the SCOBY should be discarded.

What Do I Ferment?

Almost anything can be fermented and made into a beneficial food. Fermented foods are easiest and least expensive when foods are purchased in season and made as you like. Some people ferment the vegetables that are in season. Others ferment what is on sale. Mixing and matching vegetables to ferment is beneficial, as is following tried-and-true, traditional recipes.

The best and most favored fermented foods often happen by accident, like this fermented cranberry sauce, listed below. This recipe is made in the same way cranberry sauce is made, but without heating the mixture. Just put the ingredients in the jar (cranberries, oranges, cinnamon, salt, lemon, and honey) and let the salt do the work of fermenting. It is divine as a topping for pastured pork.

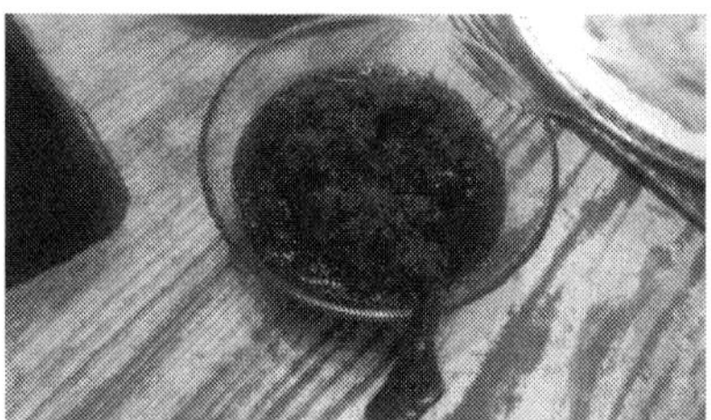

Fermented cranberry sauce is an easy dish for Thanksgiving prep, especially since it gets made at least 12 days before Thanksgiving dinner. It is another dish that can get checked off the list early, leaving you with less to do for a big holiday celebration. It keeps in the refrigerator for months — even years; realistically, it could be made in March and still be delicious on the Thanksgiving table.

This recipe is very flexible. When you take the rinds off the oranges and lemons, it is best to remove the seeds before chopping. You can use the sliced-up oranges and lemons or just the juice — it's your choice.

Honey in a ferment like this makes the product sweet; however, the honey is also fermented. Fermented honey amplifies the healing aspects of beneficial pollen. Adding liquid to honey ferments this medicinal food. It requires 19 percent liquid, which is provided by the juice from the lemons and oranges, in order to ferment. In drought years, honey contains more liquid, making a thinner and runnier honey — God's way of hydrating the bees when water is scarce. Drought year raw honey is more likely to ferment due to the higher water content.

Raw honey that is left at room temperature, which then crystallizes, has a higher potential to ferment. Higher levels of dextrose in honey will cause it to crystallize more quickly. It may contain a large or small chunk of what looks like white feathery patterns in sections, or it may have a large piece of crystallized honey.

The salt helps to ferment the food and add flavor. This cranberry sauce will be more of a sour and tart food; adding more honey will make it a sweet, sour, and tart dish.

Fermenting this dish is best done by putting the ingredients into a Mason jar, with a lid that is fingertip tight.

Set the jar on the counter under a towel or in a cabinet for 7-12 days; then refrigerate.

Fermented Cranberry Sauce

A Tangy Addition to the Thanksgiving Table

Ingredients

1 package cranberries, 12 ounces
1/2 cup local honey
3 oranges, no seeds, rinds removed
Rind from two oranges, pitch removed, cut into thin strips about an inch long
2 lemons, no seeds, rinds removed

2 teaspoons ground cinnamon
1/4 teaspoon ground clove
1 tablespoon mineral salt

Instructions

Coarse chop cranberries to desired size. Combine all ingredients into a large bowl (everything — including lemons), and let sit for 20 minutes. Pack into Mason jars, pressing down ingredients until liquid covers the top. If there is not enough liquid to cover the top, add a small amount of filtered water. Cover with the lid, fingertip tight, and let sit in a cabinet or under a towel on the countertop for 7-12 days. Refrigerate and enjoy.

Experimenting with different foods and different flavors can be a family tradition.

Remember, the FDA has no reports of anyone getting ill or dying from vegetable ferments. Meat ferments such as salmon, pork, beef, and others do contain the risk of salmonella. The process of vegetable fermentation involves a step that cannot allow growth of salmonella.

You can, however, experience die-off from vegetable ferments.

Again, probiotic vegetables can be made with just salt in a manner that is considered wild fermentation. The general ratio of salt to product is right around one tablespoon of salt per quart of vegetables and water. Some use two tablespoons of salt per quart. Too much salt will result in a salty product and will inhibit beneficial growth. Too little salt will result in kahm yeast growth, which looks like a white film floating on top.

Kahm yeast is not detrimental to your body; you just do not need a large quantity of it. Scooping it off the top is recommended.

Ferments can also be made using whey sourced from home-brewed kefir, yogurt, or sour cream.

Whey purchased from the store in bulk containers is sourced from the cheese-brewing industry. It has been heated and dehydrated. This is a dead product and should not be used in fermentation or in any other food preparation. For food to nourish you, minimal processing is best.

Whey from home-brewed dairy is used just like salt and can be substituted for salt.

The general rule of thumb in using whey is to substitute the whey for half of the salt, as laid out in *Nourishing Traditions*.[ccci]

This means that if the recipe calls for two tablespoons of salt to ferment the vegetable, you can use one tablespoon of salt and one tablespoon of whey.

If the recipe calls for three tablespoons of whey and three tablespoons of salt, you can just use six tablespoons of salt if you like.

Whey assists in speeding up the brewing process.

Traditional cultures generally use only salt for fermenting vegetables.

Vegetable fermentation is a process that happens without oxygen, an anaerobic process. If the vegetables are peeking above the brine in the jar, they are exposed to oxygen and will eventually go moldy. Traditionally, this mold is scraped off and thrown away, while the remaining product below is eaten. Remember that vegetable ferments have been made for hundreds of centuries, traveled the world on horseback and donkey, and even journeyed across oceans, sloshing back and forth with the rocking boat.

When it comes to vegetable fermentation, it is not a highly advanced skill or complicated in any way. It is simply vegetable preservation.

Weighing the vegetable down under the brine is done to prevent the oxidation and molding of the fermenting vegetable. Many different items can be used as weights to keep the vegetables below the water, including glass crock weights called crock rocks, pieces of wood, ceramic pieces, large vegetable leaves and even washed shells or stones collected from the yard.

If items from the yard or forest are used, be sure that they have not been sprayed with pesticides or used by animal walkers for the animals to relieve themselves.

Fermented Coconut Water

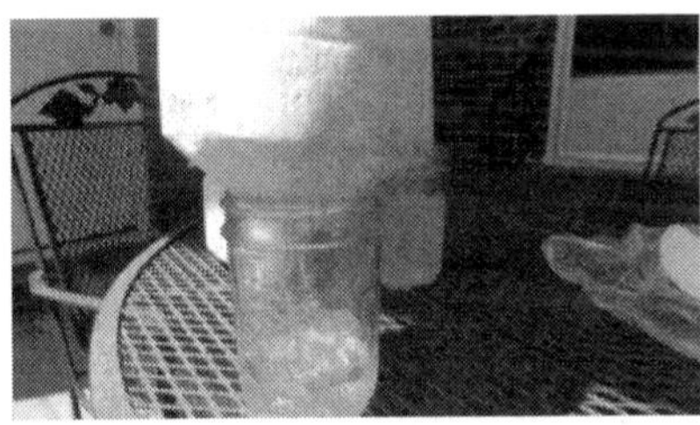

Fermented coconut water is one of the easiest probiotic drinks to make. Beginners jump into fermenting coconut water as a good introduction to fermentation. You can purchase fermented coconut water online, but it is never as good as home-brewed.

Start by buying a fresh coconut for the coconut water. The best option would be to pick a coconut from the tree yourself. Store-bought coconuts are usually sprayed with a layer of formaldehyde to keep the coconut from spoiling or discoloring during shipping and while on display in the store. This is by no means acceptable. Formaldehyde will not nourish your body in any way.

With that said, you are drilling a hole through this layer — watch for sensitivities and consider this fact if reactions other than die-off exist.

In the past, GAPS has followed the protocol of not using prepared, packaged coconut water since it is pasteurized and dead food. However, if you do not have access to coconut water from real coconuts, using packaged coconut water with no added ingredients is a viable option. It is not optimal, but it can still add tremendous benefits. Using a fresh coconut is always best.

Coconuts grow by starting off as small, green balls that advance in size until they are full-grown. At the full-grown, green coconut stage, they are filled with coconut water and a thin layer of coconut pudding on the inside wall of the nut. As the coconut matures the outer layering, the area outside the shell, called the copra, turns brown while the water inside the coconut turns into coconut meat. This meat is removed from the coconut and shredded, creating coconut flakes, which we buy in bags at the store. Left to grow and mature further, all of the water inside the coconut goes toward growing a tree by creating a sponge layer on the side of the coconut meat. This sponge layer is a delicacy. When this happens, roots sprout out of two of the eyes on the nut while a sprout grows from the third eye. This sprout will become a new palm tree.

Coconuts picked freshly from a coconut tree will have the most water. A young coconut will have a green color to the outer shell. This outer shell and the material between the outer shell and the coconut shell, the copra, will be soft. As the coconut ages on the tree, the outer green coating will age, start to grow brown spots, and eventually turn completely brown, making a hard, outer layer.

The best time to pick a coconut from the tree, when picking it for water, is when the outer shell is a vibrant green.

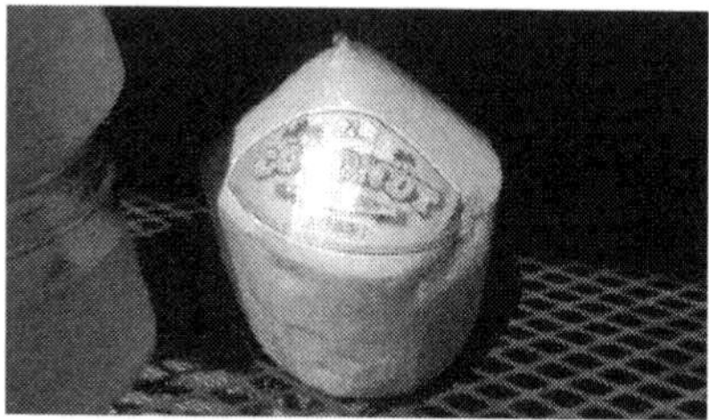

If you have no choice but to use a coconut from the store, start by removing the plastic wrap coating. Drill two holes into the top of the coconut.

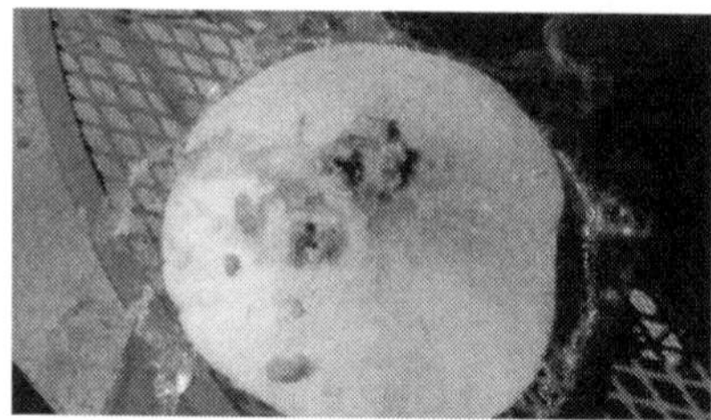

Invert the coconut over a glass to drain.

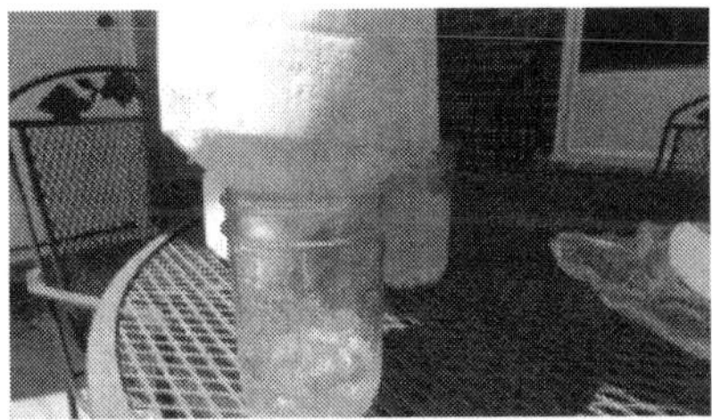

Some particles of coconut meat will fall into the glass; this is not concerning.

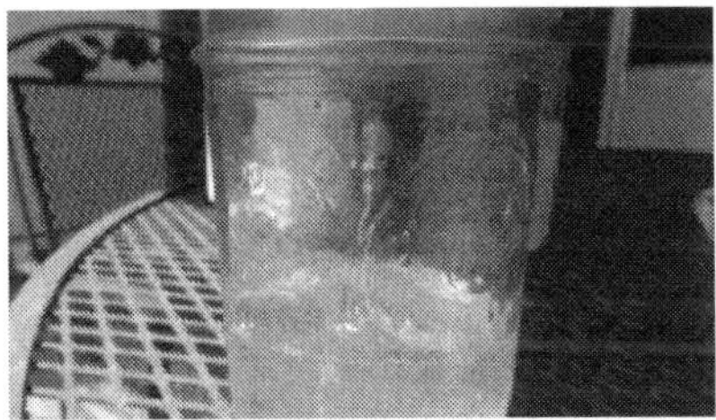

Open one of your favorite probiotic capsules, and add it to the coconut water. Stir, and let it sit on the counter for three to six days, depending on the temperature in your room, or until your desired fermented flavor is achieved.

If this product turns pink on top or throughout, it is moldy and should be discarded. Put the product in cold storage after brewing to prevent mold.

There are many ways to ferment coconut water into fermented coconut water, including using whey, probiotic capsules emptied into the coconut water, salt, or a previously fermented brine, such as kraut juice.

If using a probiotic capsule, be sure to use a probiotic that does not contain ingredients that feed pathogens. We want the cleanest and healthiest product possible.

Kefir grains added to the coconut water will create different strains, which are also highly beneficial.

To create a balanced and diverse microbiome, all methods of fermenting should be used.

Fermented Garlic

Garlic is well-known as a natural antibiotic, shows antifungal and antibacterial properties, and is a naturally testosterone-boosting food.

Making garlic into a fermented food is like putting blue tights and a red cape on a glasses-wearing newsman.

Fermenting garlic can be done with the skins left on or with the cloves peeled. The two methods result in two totally different end products. Leaving the skin on the garlic while it ferments will create a deeper, woodier, and sometimes bitter flavor.

Cloves can change color during fermentation. This happens most when using pesticide-free garlic and is normal. In fact, it is desired.

Epicurious says, "'We don't know a lot about this,' says Dr. Luke LaBorde of Penn State University's Department of Food Science. 'It's definitely enzymatic and nonenzymatic reactions occurring in the garlic, but we really don't know entirely why'." [cccii]

Some say that this is connected to the variations of different nutrients.

"The bioactivity of some natural products is increased by fermentation,"[ccciii] says *Nutrition Research*. They reported that fermented garlic protected diabetic, obese mice through the antioxidant activity of the fermented garlic vs. the unfermented garlic. The study showed remarkable liver support and anti-obesity effects.

Plant Foods for Human Nutrition, a publication of the Netherlands, reported a study on fermented garlic that showed, "Superoxide dismutase (SOD)-like activity, scavenging activity against hydrogen peroxide and the polyphenol content of the garlic extract were increased 13-[fold], more than 10-[fold], and 7-[fold], respectively, as compared with those of the control garlic extract."[ccciv]

They go on to say, "The fermented garlic is suggested to possess desirable anti-oxidative properties."[cccv] What is specifically interesting is, as they say, "Hydrogen peroxide is generated from the scavenging reaction by SOD."[cccvi]

This means that fermented garlic contains the cleansing and healing properties of hydrogen peroxide. The gut microbiome makes hydrogen peroxide naturally when it is healthy. This means that eating fermented garlic could assist in mimicking a healthy microbiome. It certainly means that it cleans the tract.

Fermented garlic powder was used in a study with 144 pigs that had just been weaned. The 5-week trial showed an increase of total tract digestibility after the use of the fermented garlic powder.[cccvii]

The Journal of Animal Physiology and Animal Nutrition reported the study, concluding that "dietary fermented garlic powder decreased the blood total cholesterol. The triglyceride concentration was decreased. Dietary fermented garlic powder can also increase the nutrient digestibility, lymphocytes and RBC concentrations, but decrease the fecal *E. coli* concentration in weaning pigs."[cccviii]

Peeled and blanched garlic was compared with unblanched garlic during fermentation, as reported by the *International Journal of Food Microbiology*. The blanched garlic was prepared by pouring boiling water over the peeled garlic for 15 minutes prior to fermentation. They reported, "The starter grew abundantly in the case of blanched garlic, producing mainly lactic acid and reaching a pH of 3.8 after 7 days, but its growth was inhibited in unblanched garlic. Ethanol and fructose, coming from enzymatic activities of the garlic, and a green pigment were formed during the fermentation of unblanched garlic, but not of blanched garlic."[cccix]

More research needs to be done to determine which is a more beneficial probiotic, blanched or unblanched.

Sometimes, when fermenting garlic, the cloves change colors, as shown above with the green pigment of the unblanched, fermented garlic.

Epicurious says, "As far as they can tell, garlic enzymes — which give it that distinct flavor — break down over time. Naturally occurring sulfur in the garlic interacts with those enzymes, occasionally turning it slightly green or blue. Sometimes the color change happens, sometimes it doesn't. Shifts in temperature, pH, and the age of the garlic can also come into play."[cccx]

Older garlic turns blue or green more frequently than fresh garlic.

The *Journal of Food Science* reported a study where they tested all 22 amino acids with garlic fermentation. They said, "Blue–green pigments are easily generated by mixing juice from heated white onions, a good source of 1-PeCSO (1-propenyl-L-cysteine sulfoxide) [which causes the] formation of thiosulfinates, 'color developers'."[cccxi]

They further concluded that "green discoloration" in crushed garlic represents a mixture of yellow and blue pigments, and that the blue color results from at least 8 pigments, depending on amino acid composition, rather than from a single blue pigment. Results indicated that amino acids other than glycine have the potential to form blue pigments."[cccxii]

The color transition is normal.

The *Journal of Agriculture and Food Industry* posted another study testing the pigmented fermented garlic saying, "Alliinase and acetic acid were required for the color formation. UV-vis spectral measurements and pH results suggest that the color formation occurs by two kinds of processes: one enzymatic and the other nonenzymatic."[cccxiii]

Some traditional cultures make what is known as black garlic, a totally different product from fermented garlic.

Black garlic is made by putting dried, unpeeled garlic in the slow cooker on the warm setting for 12-20 days without opening the lid. This is not a highly probiotic food, but it is a beneficial food. Heat reduces probiotic function.

Probably the most telling aspect of fermented garlic is its incredible power against staph and the bacteria MRSA (*Methicillin-resistant Staphylococcus aureus*). MRSA, which is specifically resistant to antibiotic use, is consistently no match for fermented garlic.

Microbiologist and Pharmaceutical Scientist says, "Unlike antibiotic drugs, garlic is very complex, containing 27 known active ingredients and dozens more that work in unknown ways. Many of these ingredients can work together synergistically inside the body in intricate ways to fight infections. The herb is highly effective against resistant MRSA bacteria because it is too complex chemically for the bacteria to become resistant. In contrast, the antibiotic drug Zyvox, which is prescribed for many MRSA cases has only one active ingredient: Linzolid."[cccxiv]

The British Journal of Biomedical Science says, "Resistance to mupirocin in MRSAs is increasing. Allicin is the main antibacterial agent isolated from garlic." They tested garlic isolates and found that "88% of clinical isolates had MBCs of 128 microg/mL, and all were killed at 256 microg/mL. Of these strains, 82% showed intermediate or full resistance to mupirocin; however, this study showed that a concentration of 500 microg/mL in an aqueous cream base was required to produce an activity equivalent to 256 microg/mL allicin liquid."[cccxv]

Fermenting garlic is one of the easiest and most potent things a person can do for his or her health.

The hardest thing about making fermented garlic is peeling the cloves. The easiest way to complete this task is to place the head of garlic on the counter top with the tip down and then press with the palm of your hand. Push down, straight into the countertop to break apart the cloves. Place the cloves in a quart or half gallon Mason jar with the lid in place. Be sure to keep about a third of the vessel filled with cloves.

They need room to hit each other.

Shake this hard. Shake it aggressively. After three to ten minutes of shaking, the cloves will be separated from their skins. Again, aggressive shaking is needed.

Fill a quart Mason jar full of garlic cloves (peeled or unpeeled, your choice), and add a tablespoon of mineral salt, such as Himalayan Pink Salt, Celtic Grey Salt, or Redmond's Real Salt. Fill the jar with filtered water, leaving an inch of headroom. Let the jar sit for a few weeks or longer. Refrigerate the product. It will gradually taste better and better over time.

Other methods of fermenting garlic have their own unique benefits.

Honey-fermented garlic is made by filling a jar with garlic cloves and covering the cloves with local honey. Put the lid on and let it sit in a corner for a month. The honey can be watered down if this is too sweet for you.

Garlic can also be placed in olive oil and left to sit, making a garlic-infused oil. Some say that using this method takes a little heating of the oil so that any potential of botulism is eradicated. Others just let it sit and count on the fact that the garlic is antibacterial, antimicrobial, and antifungal. If you choose to heat the olive oil, heat up some olive oil gently. Be sure not to heat the oil too much because that will change its molecular structure, and it will go rancid. Pour the olive oil over chopped or whole garlic. Let the mixture sit. This mixture is an excellent food.

Using a one-to-one ratio of oil to garlic (finely chopped) creates a fantastic ear infection elixir. This remedy has been used for centuries when children get glue ear or ear infections.

Fermented garlic is not the only food that attacks staph; coconut oil is also powerful against the pathogenic strain. Sally Fallon says, "Recent research, in which Mary Enig was involved, showed that the types of fats in coconut oil are the ideal treatment for the antibiotic-resistant *Staph. aureus*, which is killing so many people in our hospitals."[cccxvi]

Staph is an infection caused by a group of bacteria commonly found in hospitals. It is resistant to antibiotics; however, it cannot live in the presence of fermented garlic and fermented garlic brine. A staph infection can be fatal.

Since we have seen that fermented garlic kills pathogenic staph and MRSA, it is safe to say this may be the most necessary medicinal remedy kept in the cabinet. There are no resistant strains known to be more powerful than fermented garlic.

Most holistic practitioners who use fermented foods regularly in their practice recommend that people make fermented garlic early on in their healing journey. It is valuable to have on hand in emergencies.

Please note that if there is a health issue, visiting your primary care physician is recommended. If there is an emergency, calling 911 or going to the local emergency room is recommended.

Some say that they use peeled, bagged garlic to make fermented garlic. They do this because they know that they will not take the time to peel garlic with every meal or peel the garlic to make fermented garlic. What we currently know, as stated previously, is that fermenting foods eats up the pesticides, rendering conventional garlic safe to use, even though it is not as beneficial as organic garlic.

Probiotic Pickles

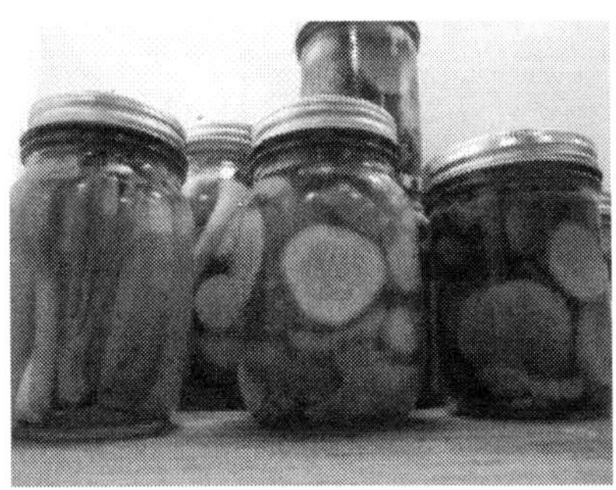

When cucumbers are abundant in the garden, probiotic pickles are a popular choice. These GAPS-approved pickles are a fermented vegetable, high in beneficial digestive aspects.

The base recipe for a quart size jar of pickles is:

2 oak leaves or grape leaves (more may be used if desired)
Cucumbers (be sure to cut off the flower end as it contains enzymes that make wimpy pickles)
Chopped green onions or quartered white onions
1 tablespoon mustard seed
1 teaspoon dill, preferably fresh
Onion and garlic, chopped or sliced to your liking
1 tablespoon mineral salt
Adding one tablespoon of organic sugar or local honey is optional. If you are on GAPS, honey should be used.

Pack all of the ingredients in the quart jar with an oak leaf on the bottom and an oak leaf on the top. Be sure to leave one inch of headroom at the top so that the brine doesn't bubble over and leak during the fermentation process.

Pickles may be sliced in any manner you desire for eating. Again, for crisper pickles, be sure to put one oak leaf on the bottom of the jar; then pack in the other ingredients, and place the second oak leaf on the top. Fill the jar with filtered water. Put the lid on the jar and leave it on the counter for 3 days; then refrigerate.

This recipe is also delicious with ginger added.

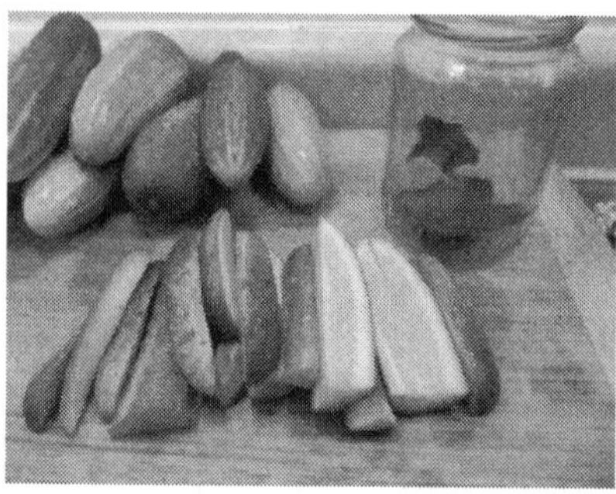

Slice the cucumbers in a way that leaves one inch of headroom above the cucumbers.

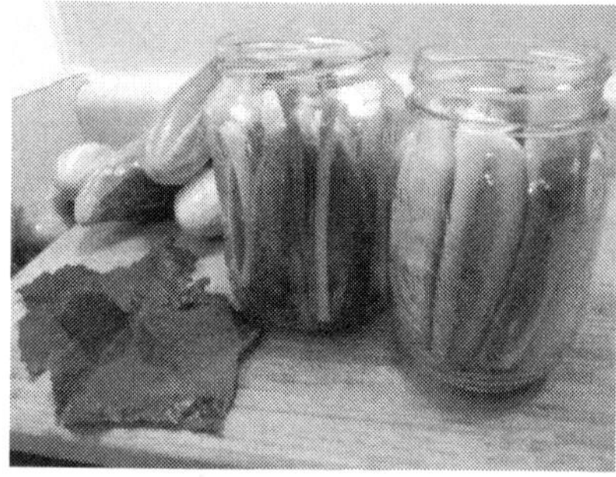

The oak leaf can be substituted with a grape leaf or any other leaf that contains tannins.

Some probiotic foods are stronger than others or have beneficial strains that are more common in the intestinal tract, even in those with deeper intestinal damage. For most people, probiotic pickles, dilly carrots, fermented asparagus, fermented green beans, and the like, are easier starting places than kraut juice or kefir.

Anything can be added to probiotic pickles to add new flavor to the batch. Each additional seasoning or vegetable added to the ferment will introduce a whole new host of variable beneficial strains. When making pickles, spicy red pepper flakes can be added for heat. Different peppers create different beneficial strains in the ferment; this includes sweet peppers as well as hot peppers. Adding shaved carrot or beets also creates various strains to benefit the microbiome.

The goal is variety. It would be a mistake to make probiotic pickles one way and to consistently eat them in only that way. Every time we change the recipe, the probiotic strains change, feeding different beneficial bacteria in the microbiome. This variety creates a level of balance as well as strength.

In this way, it is also better to use salt as a starter one time, whey from kefir the next, then whey from yogurt or sour cream, a probiotic capsule, kefir grains, or a starter packet – creating a little difference in the beneficial strains with each batch. The goal is to create balance through many different strains.

Diversity is key.

Common Probiotic Strains

Many strains of good and bad microbes fill the intestinal tract. Each has a purpose. Each can grow out of control if not kept in check with balance.

When there is damage, rebuilding is possible. Knowing where to attack is important for most.

Following studies on these most popular species can help guide you.

Bacteroides

> *Current Protocols in Microbiology* says, "They are the predominant indigenous bacterial species in the human intestinal tract, where they play an important role in the normal physiology of the host, but they can also be significant opportunistic pathogens."[cccxvii]
>
> *Cellular Microbiology* says Bacteroides assists in the processes that lead to the formation of tight junctions in the intestinal tract. This is the prevention of Intestinal Permeability.[cccxviii]
>
> When Bacteroides is low, the potential for Intestinal Permeability is high. Intestinal Permeability, Leaky Gut, leads to autoimmune disease.

Bifidobacterium

> The *Journal of Pediatric Gastroenterology and Nutrition* says that *Bifidobacteria* reduces the prevalence of neonatal necrotizing enterocolitis, a disease which primarily affects premature infants. This disease is calculated as a devastating disease where the intestinal wall is invaded with bacteria, causing infections and inflammation. Left unchecked, it can destroy the intestinal tract.[cccxix]

Medline Plus shows that *Bifidobacteria*, specifically from fermented milk products, assists with constipation, *H. pylori*, IBS, ulcerative colitis, pouchitis, eczema, yeast infections, cold, flu, reducing flu-like symptoms in children attending day-care centers, breast pain (mastitis), hepatitis, lactose intolerance, mumps, Lyme disease, cancer, boosting the immune system, lowering cholesterol, and aiding in the bowel infection called necrotizing enterocolitis.[cccxx]

Enterococcus faecium

The American Journal of Clinical Nutrition says that *E. faecium* shortened the effects and duration of stomach and intestinal inflammation. Their findings recommend using *E. faecium* from fermented milk products to treat attention deficit disorder (ADD).[cccxxi]

Lactobacillus

Lactobacillus is a bacterium which comes in many strains. It should dominate the intestinal tract.

Applied and Environmental Microbiology says that Lactobacillus has many beneficial properties, including the ability to "adhere to cells; exclude or reduce pathogenic adherence; persist and multiply; produce acids, hydrogen peroxide, and bacteriocins antagonistic to pathogen growth; resist vaginal microbicides, including spermicides; be safe and therefore noninvasive, noncarcinogenic, and nonpathogenic; and coaggregate and form a normal, balanced flora."[cccxxii]

Lactobacillus rhamnosus, L. reuteri, L. acidophilus, L. fermentum, L. rhamnosus, L. plantarum, L. casei and L. johnsonii are among the most popular but certainly are not the only beneficial strains.

Lactobacillus rhamnosus

The American Journal of Clinical Nutrition says that *L. rhamnosus* shortens the duration of travelers' diarrhea as well as diarrhea in infants caused by rotavirus enteritis. It is also thought to shorten gastroenteritis, inflammation of the stomach and intestines resulting from bacteria or a virus. *Lactobacillus rhamnosus* is found in fermented milk products.[cccxxiii]

Allergies, Asthma & Clinical Immunology reported a study using mice with induced allergies to milk products. The study showed that fermented milk product containing *Lactobacillus rhamnosus* reduced the cow's milk allergy.[cccxxiv]

In fact, *L. rhamnosus* has been found to assist in eliminating multiple allergies including anaphylaxis to products such as peanuts, nuts and eggs.

The Journal of Allergy and Clinical Immunology reported a study on the use of *L. rhamnosus* enabling those studied to walk away from peanut anaphylaxis (peanut allergies).[cccxxv]

Using this method, when anaphylaxis exists, should only be done under the close care and observation of a qualified practitioner. Rebuilding can be done; however, if done too quickly or incorrectly, it can cause severe problems, especially for those who have anaphylaxis.

The Journal of Medical Microbiology showed that *L. rhamnosus* decreased inflammation of the stomach and intestines in acute stages.[cccxxvi]

Saccharomyces boulardii

The *American Journal of Clinical Nutrition* reported a study, saying, "Use *S. boulardii* to prevent further recurrence of relapsing diarrhea because of *C. difficile*." *Clostridium difficile* diarrhea was shut down in the presence of *S. boulardii*.[cccxxvii]

Therapeutic Advances in Gastroenterology reported a study showing that *S. boulardii* reduced persistent and acute diarrhea, traveler's diarrhea, *H. pylori*, and *C. diff* infection; brought about fewer relapses for those with Crohn's disease; prevented early ulcerative colitis flares; assisted with IBS; and showed a beneficial effect on protozoan infections of amebiasis, giardiasis and infection with *Blastocystis hominis*.[cccxxviii]

Using Fermented Foods to Their Fullest Potential

As discussed, different probiotic foods have different benefits.

Making sauerkraut will provide a host of beneficial strains. Adding a carrot to that same sauerkraut will change up the whole structure and add different benefits through different probiotic strains.

Adding a carrot, an onion, celery, garlic, and red pepper flakes to that same sauerkraut mix feeds and adds a whole different host of beneficial strains.

Changing up fermented foods is beneficial in this manner. At the same time, listening to what your body needs and feeding it the strains it desires, as well as the strains that are the antithesis to the pathogenic strain or strains present, is optimal.

Eating fermented beans, kimchi, kefir, kvass, sour cream, yogurt, curtido, probiotic pickles, gari (pickled ginger), sauerkraut, kraut juice, sourdough, and all of the other fermented foods will assist in rebuilding the microbiome.

Neurotransmitters are set in motion by different strains.

Psychology Today says, "*Lactobacillus* and *Bifidobacterium* species are known to produce GABA. *Escherichia, Bacillus*, and *Saccharomyces* produce norepinephrine. *Candida*, *Streptococcus*, *Escherichia*, and *Enterococcus* produce serotonin. *Bacillus* and *Serratia* produce dopamine, and *Lactobacillus* species produce acetylcholine."[cccxxix]

The *British Journal of Nutrition* reported a study using rats and human volunteers. They reported findings showing that probiotics with *Lactobacillus helveticus* and *Bifidobacterium longum* "significantly reduced anxiety-like behavior in rats and alleviated psychological distress in volunteers." There was also a remarkable improvement in depression, anger, multiple symptoms that had no apparent cause, hostility, hospital anxiety, or depression.[cccxxx]

As explained, kefir is highly beneficial for pathogenic streptococcal strains, which present as PANDAS symptoms including tics, obsessive compulsive behaviors, hyperactivity, jerky movements, ADHD symptoms, anxiety, separation anxiety, mood changes, bed wetting, foul smelling urine, trouble voiding, joint pain, or altered fine motor skills. It also assists in degrading pesticides within the body.

As previously mentioned, fermented garlic has proven beneficial with yeast overgrowth, brain fog, forgetfulness, pink eye, rashes, MRSA, and staph.

Kombucha assists the liver with processing fat and supports the liver and kidneys.

Home brewed yogurt has beneficial strains that combat a yeast infection, as does kombucha and kefir.

Each probiotic is going to help in its own way. Finding out what works best for your own microbiome is optimal.

As previously stated with fermented coconut water, a probiotic capsule can be added to ferment foods, just as salt and whey can be added. This method of brewing a probiotic is very young in the investigation stages. In an interview with Dr. Mercola, Sandor Katz said he didn't believe adding a probiotic to a ferment would change the outcome; it changed the pH earlier in the fermentation process.

Some think that if you add a probiotic to the ferment, it creates those dominant strains in the end result.

This belief has not been thoroughly studied enough to have definitive results.

For example, some have added powdered starter cultures, with isolated strains, to a vegetable ferment, saying that those specific strains are dominant in that fermentation.

This has not shown the same results in home fermentation products.

For example, when we take a person who is deficient in specific strains, they will have a massive die-off response from just one drop of the probiotic containing those strains; therefore, if we take that probiotic and add it to a batch of sauerkraut, it stands to reason that the batch of sauerkraut should be dominated with that strain that made the person have the massive die-off.

Clinically, this doesn't prove to be true.

Clinically, tracking die-off responses, sauerkraut will become what sauerkraut is, no matter what we add.

When a specific probiotic creates a highly sensitive response, with enormous die-off from one drop, it doesn't have the same resulting die-off from that fermentation. Instead, the die-off has been shown to be the same, with or without the inoculation from the sensitive strain. The die-off tolerance has been shown to be the same each time.

Applied and Environmental Microbiology reported a study performed with fermentation of Spanish green olives testing this exact scenario. They reported, "In the ferment inoculated with *L. plantarum* the population of this strain did not predominate but simply rose and fell as one component in the natural succession of eight Lactobacillus strains."[cccxxxi]

This result is exactly what Sandor Katz explained in his interview with Dr. Mercola. The addition of a specific probiotic strain will change the pH of the fermented food earlier, but in the end, the product is the same, with or without the specific isolated strains. He calls this "wild fermentation" and wrote a book on the topic of the same name — *Wild Fermentation*. The vegetables will do what they are supposed to do, with or without an added starter culture aiming to produce a product high in those strains.

Donna Gates has been inoculating ferments at her company, Body Ecology, with isolated strains and getting what she says are enormous results in the strains inoculating the product. This means that a specific strain like *Lactobacillus rhamnosus* was added to sauerkraut, hoping to produce a sauerkraut product higher in *Lactobacillus rhamnosus*.

An email request to her company asking for more information regarding the specific strain count after using that specific probiotic inoculation received this answer:

> Thank you for reaching out. This was internal testing on different culture combinations done with our supplier, and we aren't able to give out the details as they are proprietary.
>
> Warm Regards,
>
> Donald
>
> Body Ecology

Another email was sent, clarifying that proprietary information was not desired; merely the count of the resulting probiotic strains with a specific culture strain starter was being requested.

There was no reply.

Probiotics are a supplement, meaning that they are part of a self-regulated industry. There is no way to verify that the probiotic count on the bottle of a product is the same as the probiotic count of actual capsules. The same is true for the beneficial strains said to be in each product.

Clinically, we see the same die-off from the same vegetables. Clinically, we see that variety can be achieved through probiotic foods. The goal is diversity and variety. Food-based probiotics, as well as commercial probiotics, offer a fantastic method of consistency and feeding elements.

The choice is in the consumer's hands.

Commercial Probiotics

Strong, therapeutic probiotics are often a part of healing a damaged gut.

For those with the most damaged guts, recommended probiotics assist in healing the gut.

Other probiotics, with ingredients that are not GAPS-compliant, do the exact opposite. Pathogen-feeding ingredients feed the pathogens, whether they are found in food or in supplements.

Dr. Natasha Campbell-McBride said at the 2012 Wise Traditions Conference in London, "GAPS diet is very rich in nutrition. You will get all your nutrition, all your vitamins, all your minerals from food. A handful of supplements are very helpful, particularly at the beginning. The probiotic market is full of various brands. The majority of them are prophylactic. They are designed for healthy people to boost themselves a little bit, and they don't make a huge difference in the body."[cccxxxii]

An effective probiotic, at a dosage specific to that person, is classified as a therapeutic strength probiotic. Once the therapeutic dose is reached, the protocol while on GAPS is to hold the therapeutic dosage for a certain length of time, individual to that person — usually six months.

Dr. Natasha says, "Strong therapeutic probiotics, when they come into your gut, will start killing Clostridium, killing Protells, killing Staphylococcus and Streptococcus, and killing other pathogens. When these creatures die, they release toxins which make your child autistic or hyperactive or gives him epilepsy or multiple sclerosis, or gives you arthritis, migraine headaches, or something else. This reaction is called a die-off reaction."[cccxxxiii]

These symptoms are specific to each person.

The pathogens living in the gut are living beings, exhaling and sloughing off dead cells and releasing their toxic gases. The toxic gases from these pathogens that give your original symptoms are the same toxic gases released when the pathogens die – releasing the toxic gases into the bloodstream and causing the same symptoms as the original illness.

When a person takes a probiotic with strains they are weak in, it can cause the person to say, "We can't tolerate this!"

This die-off causes some people to flee from the very thing that is healing. Reactions like this are the body speaking to you, telling you what it needs. Discontinuing the probiotic altogether may or may not be the right decision. Going more slowly may be more fitting; however, pathogen feeders in the probiotics are a definite reason to abort. Food probiotics ensure cofactors for absorption and ensure no pathogen feeding ingredients.

On the GAPS protocol, rebuilding is done methodically.

Once a probiotic is introduced — at the smallest amount without a die-off response — gradually increase the dose until the therapeutic strength is reached. Some people need to open a probiotic capsule and take what fits on the tip of a pin head to start. Each person's starting point is very bio-individual.

Wherever you start, you start.

If nothing happens from the dose after a couple of days, increase or even double the amount. The protocol is to continue this method until the therapeutic dose is reached.

Staying on the therapeutic dose for a few months enables and encourages healthy bacteria to kill off the pathogenic bacteria and allow homeostasis to establish a foothold.

Consuming probiotics on an empty stomach can diminish the probiotic aspect since the stomach acid damages some of the beneficial bacteria.

Taking probiotics at the end of the meal or after drinking a full glass of water is optimal for beneficial bacteria.

The probiotics listed below are those recommended for the most damaged guts and are all considered therapeutic strength at your individual dosage. These are the cleaner therapeutic probiotics with the least potential to feed pathogens.

Prescript Assist contains 29 strains of microflora from soil-based organisms and is shelf-stable, not needing refrigeration. It is considered both a prebiotic and probiotic. The manufacturer explains that probiotic bacteria are encompassed in a seed-like barrier, which ensures that the probiotic bacteria makes it through the stomach and into the intestines with over 95% effectiveness. This same protective barrier allows for a two-year shelf life. The manufacturer recommends taking this product with meals.[cccxxxiv]

Many practitioners see great results using Prescript Assist and prefer it over others. Many clients respond favorably. In addition, soil-based organisms are just like all other probiotics: they are transient. This means that the probiotics pass through the tract, they don't reside indefinitely in the tract. Soil- based organisms, however, set up little colonies in the tract, where they stay a bit longer than others.

Gut Pro has eight strains; however, it does not contain D-lactate, which causes acidosis in some people. The *L. plantarum* in GutPro reverses acidosis. D-lactic acidosis occurs with microbiome damage, in which state the body cannot properly metabolize excess D-lactate.

Biokult is considered the gold standard of probiotics for GAPS people. Each person's gut flora is missing certain strains, which may not necessarily be in Biokult. Choosing a probiotic is a very individual situation. Dr. McBride helped formulate the original Biokult product, making it specifically geared towards those patients with GAPS damaged guts. The manufacturer uses food sources in which they grow strains, then scrape the strains off the top and discard the food source. Two of the food sources are soya and milk. Personal correspondence with the manufacturer reveals this about the process: "The soya and other food sources are filtered out and discarded. It goes through a filtration process a number of times. This is a standard process used by most probiotic fermentation companies."[cccxxxv] Biokult uses organic food sources that are non-GMO and, at the time of print, does not use corn.

Living Streams is a liquid that, according to the manufacturer, "is NOT a full spectrum probiotic, although it does contain the original bacteri[a] which produced the Living Streams Probiotic™ solution, and grow in the intestinal area, which is many times as powerful as any probiotic product can produce in the body naturally."[cccxxxvi]

LS Derma Gold is a paracasei flora specific liquid probiotic and is designed to be applied directly to the skin for absorption. One drop is the application dosage. The manufacturer says their products "can be used effectively by applying to the skin or be taken by mouth. You can safely use them in the eyes, ears, nose, lungs, vaginally and rectally."[cccxxxvii]

Custom Probiotics contains 2 strains, totaling 50 billion microorganisms in each pill, and requires refrigeration. This product should be refrigerated as soon as it is received.

Klaire Labs **Lactoprime Plus** contains 13 strains and 25 Billion CFUs. This product requires refrigeration.

HMF Multistrain Probiotics, and the whole HMF brand of products, is of therapeutic strength and, at the time of publication, clean for GAPS folks. Each capsule contains 15 billion CFU from 16 different strains. If taken in powder form, it is best to stir it into a bit of yogurt so that it does not stick to the roof of the mouth or to the teeth.

Body Biotics contains coveted soil-based organisms in addition to the traditional probiotic strains.

Home-fermented foods, however, may exceed all commercial probiotic brands in CFUs and bio-availablility. Early test results are showing these results in every fermented food tested, to date.

Sometimes, the liver needs support to assist with detoxing and properly cleaning out channels. PEKANA Basic Detox & Drainage Kit has been shown to assist in very stubborn cases. This is not recommended for GAPS patients unless they have been on the program for two years and are still suffering from a struggling liver.

The homeopathic remedy China 200, otherwise known as Cinchona (China) Officinalis 200, which can be ordered online by the general public from ABC Homeopathy, is highly effective for supporting and clearing the liver. After roughly eight consecutive doses of China 200 (four drops under the tongue, every hour), many say that they see liver flukes in their bowel movement, and then baby liver flukes an hour later.

Liver flukes look like portabella mushrooms that were not chewed well, with tiny tails. Baby liver flukes look like rolled up tomato skins. When liver flukes are passed like this, most folks say that the dark circles under their eyes fade.

Milk thistle seed, used as a hot medicinal tea to support the liver, steeped for 10 to 15 minutes, is highly effective for liver support. Milk thistle seed contains an element known as silymerin, which is an antioxidant which is considered extremely potent, as well as an effective anti-inflammatory. It is so strong that it has been shown to support remediating cirrhosis of the liver. The homeopathic remedy carduus marianus (also in 200C) shows phenomenal support when used with China. Carduus marianus is the homeopathic remedy from milk thistle seed.

Dandelion root granules support the liver in a superior manner. Simmered dandelion root tastes like coffee and is a good substitute that does not strip the adrenals. The support of the liver from dandelion root granules is favored over many other support methods.

Coffee enemas are highly effective for liver support for adults but are not recommended for children.

The chanca piedra tree is nicknamed The Stone Breaker, as it is known to break up gallstones made in the liver and stored in the gallbladder. Using chanca piedra as a tea turns gallstones into sludge, allowing them to pass easily. Chanca piedra can be used as a hot medicinal tea, as well as in a coffee enema, to turn stones to sludge. Most medicinal teas use the ratio of one teaspoon of dried medicinal herb to one cup of water, made into a tea. For chanca piedra, many folks use more, such as one tablespoon of dried medicinal herb to one cup of water. Drinking chanca piedra tea and then doing an enema is reported by many to remove gallstone sludge.

Any manufacturer, at any time, can change the way a product is made, rendering this list obsolete or deficient. Products are frequently evaluated for profit and loss.

The supplement industry is self-regulated.

This means that supplement products are determined safe and effective by the same company that made the supplement.

The company making the product says the ingredients are fine for human consumption; however, that may not be the case.

Beware of Fillers, Additives, Anti-caking Agents and Others

Many people who are intolerant of these probiotic products are actually responding to the prebiotics, which contain inulin. This practice of using prebiotics, however, does not have a consensus among doctors. Many doctors say no, prebiotics are bad. Others say they are the only way to go.

Clinically, we see that those with the deepest microbiome damage cannot tolerate any ingredient that feeds pathogens.

The British Journal of Nutrition says this about these prebiotics: "Through fermentation in the large intestine, prebiotic carbohydrates yield short-chain fatty acids, stimulate the growth of many bacterial species [*sic*] in addition to the selective effects on lactobacilli and bifidobacteria, they can also produce gas. Prebiotic carbohydrates clearly have significant and distinctive physiological effects in the human large intestine, and on the basis of this it is likely that they will ultimately be shown to be beneficial to health."[cccxxxviii]

Prebiotics are put into probiotics, supposedly, for the purpose of feeding bacteria which generally aggravates SIBO patients as well as those with deeper microbiome damage. The most common ingredients used in prebiotics are potato starch and chicory root, inulin. This creates a problem in the damaged microbiome.

Potato starch is the perfect example of an added ingredient to a commercial probiotic.

Dr. Natasha says that chicory root and potato starch are not to be used in patients with intestinal issues as they feed pathogens. Chicory root is highly processed.[cccxxxix]

This changes the digestibility of the product.

Products that contain inulin that do not cause intestinal upset are apple skins, bananas, onions, and garlic – all of which are GAPS-approved for healing intestinal damage.

Eating chicory root is not the same as using chicory root in tea, which Dr. Natasha does approve, as noted in the book *GAPS, Stage by Stage, with Recipes*.

The reason for this discrepancy is fiber. McBride says that people with this type of gut damage cannot digest this fiber.

Many products like Prebiotin contain oligofructose enriched inulin, a processed sugar that feeds pathogens that cause the problem. It is not GAPS-approved for healing the damaged gut.

Healing the situation of pathogen overgrowth should not come from adding more processed sugar foods, but instead, should be done through real probiotic foods and nutrient-dense foods. This could be done effectively through probiotic kraut juice made with the inulin-containing vegetables such as the apple skins, bananas, onions, and garlic, as tolerated.

The GAPS probiotic Biokult contains *Bacillus subtilis*, a specific strain that assists in repairing this situation.

For those with deeper gut damage, prebiotics do not prove beneficial, as they feed both the good strains and the bad strains equally.

If you suffer from pathogenic overgrowth, you could be feeding the pathogens.

As previously mentioned, ingredients are often added to supplements for many reasons, the top of which is usually financial gain. This financial gain can come in the form of longer shelf life or less product and more filler in the capsule, allowing for more profit.

Often, supplements and their fillers cause inflammation in a sensitive system. This is seen clinically all the time.

Some of the most common pathogen-feeding ingredients, as previously shown, are xylitol, mannitol or other sugar alcohols, synthetic sweeteners, potato starch, rice flour, sodium starch glycolate (a starch generally made from wheat, corn, rice, or potato, a free-flowing powder), yellow 5 and other color additives, anti-caking agents, free flowing agents, chicory root, microcrystalline cellulose, magnesium stearate, silica, silicon dioxide, and others.

Another very important factor is the sensitivity of the product in the capsule.

Probiotic foods are alive.

Probiotics in capsule form do not have the same properties as probiotic foods. Many factors need to be considered, including shelf stability, heat in shipping, filler ingredients, and others.

Dr. Natasha says, "Supplements on GAPS are food. Fillers and binders interfere with healing of the gut."[cccxl]

She recommends an effective probiotic but is very clear, saying, "I have many people who cannot afford supplements; they do very well on just fermented food. The process of fermentation produces many enzymes."[cccxli]

Regarding prebiotics, Dr. McBride said, "Prebiotics, just like fiber and starch, feed the good and bad equally. They cause a lot of gas. I do not recommend them."[cccxlii]

Supporting the body can be done best by reducing inflammation and not adding chemicals, additives, or fillers into the system.

It is also important to be wary of products that give a specific bacteria count "at the time of manufacture," as the probiotic count will decline during shipping and the time on the shelf.

Neurologist and medical doctor, David Perlmutter says, "You need at least five grams of them to make an impact — way more than the one-quarter gram that fits in a probiotic capsule. At these levels, it's just marketing hype."[cccxliii]

A post on Nourishing Plot listed specific, commercially made probiotics. The list was an effort to show consumers the products containing the ingredients that feed the pathogens, which should be avoided. This post was taken down after Nourishing Plot received a phone call from the CEO of a well-known supplement company. His probiotic was listed as containing ingredients that feed the pathogens. The post was taken down after the 35-minute-long phone call that contained many threats.

The CEO said, "I will ruin you. Just you wait! You don't know what the (expletive) you're talking about! Do you know how many of the most intelligent microbiologists I have working on this? You don't know (expletive). I will sue you! I will take you down! You're a (expletive) moron to say what you say, that ingredients cause harm! You take that down, or I'm coming after you! You don't know who you're (expletive) with!"

After asking for his name again, he said, "You (expletive) print my (expletive) name, and I'll (expletive) cause you a whole lot of hurt. Try me! You just try me!"

This sort of treatment is not ethical, not fair, and not appropriate, but in today's economy it is not plausible to defend yourself. Free speech or not, the cost of legally defending yourself is not financially wise.

Still, people are hoping the magic pill will heal them.

One of the bigger problems is that ingredients are not beneficial or true to the listing label.

"The FDA is doing little to ensure that all the safe and efficacious products that could come to the market are allowed to do so," says *Toxicology*. "The Dietary Supplement Health and Education Act (DSHEA) was the product of a compromise with a lower threshold for demonstration of safety (reasonable *expectation* of no harm) that would be met by consumer self-policing and assumption of some risk. FDA has thwarted this effort by raising the bar for New Dietary Ingredient Notifications (NDIN) to what appears to be the higher threshold for the safety of food ingredients (reasonable *certainty* of no harm) —FDA apparently sees these two safety thresholds as a distinction without a difference."[cccxliv]

They go on to say, "As a result, increasing numbers of dietary supplement manufacturers, unwilling to gamble the future of their products to a system that provides little hope for the FDA's response of 'no objection', have committed the additional resources necessary to obtain Generally Recognized as Safe (GRAS) status for their supplements."

JAMA Internal Medicine says this is a conflict of interest; "the lack of independent review in GRAS determinations raises concerns about the integrity of the process and whether it ensures the safety of the food supply, particularly in instances where the manufacturer does not notify the FDA of the determination."[cccxlv]

Environmental Health Perspectives says, "Castoreum, a substance used to augment some strawberry and vanilla flavorings, comes from 'rendered beaver anal gland.' Vegans were outraged to learn that Starbucks used cochineal extract, a color additive derived from insect shells, to dye their strawberry Frappuccino® drinks."[cccxlvi]

The US Government Accountability Office says, "There are substances in the food supply that are unknown to the FDA. In 2010 the Government Accountability Office (GAO) concluded that a "growing number of substances … may effectively be excluded from federal oversight."[cccxlvii]

This becomes a problem when food intolerances are present. When the microbiome is imbalanced, damaged, and prolifically occupied by pathogens, this problem is exponentially exacerbated. Those with Intestinal Permeability, Leaky Gut, suffer from these ingredients to a heavier degree because the ingredients enter the bloodstream and potentially cause worse damage.

California Healthline says, "An FDA examination of 85 companies 'of all sizes' found that 25% did not list all the raw ingredients in their products on the product labels. In addition, only 'slightly more than half' of the companies checked their products to ensure that all of the ingredients were accurately reflected on the labels."[cccxlviii]

Specifically, they go on to say, "The FDA currently requires companies to list all of a product's ingredients but allow[s] 'trace amounts' of 'natural' ingredients to be omitted."

Changing government regulations on these restrictions is expected to take years.

Wood Pulp or Cotton in Your Supplements

Cellulose is used as a binder or filler in capsules and tablets.

The EFSA Journal described the process in detail after The European Commission received a request for safety analysis. They said, "Ethyl cellulose is the ethyl ether of cellulose. Ethyl cellulose is prepared from wood pulp or cotton with alkali and ethylation of the alkali treated cellulose with ethyl chloride."[cccxlix] They said that no specific studies are known regarding this product.

A study on 80 rats lasting over eight months in 1963 showed no visible adverse effects with a diet of 1.2 percent ethyl cellulose. No other conclusions were made. They concluded, "The panel considers that during the manufacturing process, the steaming and drying steps would remove volatile residues."[cccl] Their assumptions were that the ethyl cellulose passes right through the intestinal tract "essentially unchanged. Adverse side effects are unlikely."[cccli]

However, the fact remains: cotton is not food.

If it's not food, don't put it in your mouth.

Cotton is one of the top-ranked GMO products worldwide. GMO products contain Glyphosate, which works as an antibiotic in your body.

It makes no sense to take a probiotic with an antibiotic in it, especially when it carries a high-ticket value.

Wood pulp is not food. If it's not food, don't put it in your mouth.

When you find the right probiotic for you, the one that contains strains you do not have or are weak in, the die-off will be extremely noticeable. Even one drop under the tongue can cause such severe die-off that it produces symptoms like sinus pain, cold-like symptoms, flu-like symptoms, or even a sinus headache with waves of nasal crud, as well as many other symptoms like diarrhea, joint pain, etc. This die-off can be the worst healing crisis you ever experience, including severe swollen sinuses that create an unbearable headache. In addition, it can inflame a nerve going to a tooth, which can then shoot pain through your whole head and down your neck.

Some die-off is so extreme that it renders a person unable to leave his or her bed.

Some feel sloshing liquid in their head. For others, pathogenic bacteria can inflame the intestinal tract and cause a hernia, an overgrowth of pathogenic gases in the intestinal tract pushing out the intestines in a weak spot. Tooth pain can be so bad that it can prevent sleep. A urinary tract infection (UTI) can develop from pathogenic toxins trying to escape. If the body can not eliminate these pathogens quickly enough, the downward spiral begins. The accumulation of toxins and pathogenic bacteria quickly eats through the mucosal lining of the bladder, and the pathogens cause a urinary tract infection.

For some, all of these symptoms occur simultaneously.

This does not mean that everyone will have the same enormous die-off from this probiotic. It does suggest the body's weakness in the strains represented in this probiotic.

It takes a lot of searching to find supplement products that are clean and unadulterated, with no added ingredients, fillers, binders, or free-flowing agents. These extra ingredients contained in products could be damaging your body, making your health decline. Our bodies are meant to be nourished with food, not filled with chemicals or non-food ingredients. When pipes are filled with something other than liquid, they clog. In addition, we don't know what these ingredients do to our detox pathways. We do know that when "canaries in the coalmine," those who are highly sensitive to non-food ingredients, remove these ingredients from their intake, they get better. This leads us to believe that the fewer non-food ingredients we put in, the healthier we will be.

If the body is busy fighting toxins, it cannot fight off the common cold or pollen and dog dander. The system is overworked and begins to shut down, presenting as diseased.

When we eliminate these toxins from the body, it can function as it should.

A good rule to follow is this: If it's not food, don't put it in your mouth.

Sand in Your Supplements

One common ingredient, silica, is an obvious example of an additive in supplements; silicone dioxide, silicon, and others, fall from the same source.

Clinical Reviews in Food Science Nutrition says, "Traditionally, silicas have had a broad spectra of product usage including such areas as viscosity control agents in inks, paints, corrosion-resistant coatings, etc.[,] and as excipients in pharmaceuticals and cosmetics. In the food industry, the most important application has been as an anticaking agent in powdered mixes, seasonings, and coffee whiteners."[ccclii]

They go on to say, "Amorphous silica has multifunctional properties that would allow it to act as a viscosity control agent, emulsion stabilizer, suspension and dispersion agent, desiccant, etc."[cccliii]

There must be a reason to add an ingredient to a product. The real question remains: "What does it really do to the body?"[cccliv]

Akzo Nobel, a company of over 4,000 scientists, says, "Silica is another name for silicon oxides – the most prevalent type being SiO2. It can be found in nature in crystalline form (as quartz sand), and it is the most abundant component of the earth's crust. Amorphous silica, on the other hand, is industrially manufactured in a variety of forms – including silica gels, precipitated silica, fumed silica, and colloidal silica."[ccclv]

They describe silica as sand, opal, and flint.[ccclvi]

Akzo Nobel considers itself to be from "a pioneering heritage which has created scientific breakthroughs in paints, plastics and chemistry, thanks in no small part to Alfred Nobel, one of our founding fathers."[ccclvii]

Critical Reviews in Food Science Nutrition puts it bluntly: "the utilization of silicas in these potential applications, however, has not been undertaken, partially because of the limited knowledge of their physiochemical interactions with other food components and partially due to their controversial status from a toxicological point of view."[ccclviii]

Yet, we are ingesting it in supplements, taken with food.

Life Sciences says that silica leaches into lymph nodes.[ccclix]

They further added, "Through magnetic resonance spectroscopy and atomic emission spectroscopy, silicon compounds were found in the blood of some women with silicone breast implants; silicone and silica have also been found in (the) liver. Well-publicized case reports have raised significant concerns regarding an association between implants and systemic disease."[ccclx]

The European Union says, "Silica is commonly found in nature as sand. Silica exists in many different forms that can be crystalline as well as non-crystalline (amorphous)."[ccclxi]

Diatomaceous Earth is a form of silica, in the natural form (non-crystalline) derived from amorphous silica. This product has been used traditionally in many societies as a natural dewormer and antiparasitic in humans, farm animals, and pets.

Crystalline silica is a different story. The European Union states that it is "hard, chemically inert and has a high melting point. These are valued/important properties in various industrial uses."[ccclxii]

Quartz is a crystalline silica.

When a product lists a silica as an ingredient, we really don't know what exact form it is. It could very well be Food Grade Diatomaceous Earth, a healthy product used to cleanse the body of toxins and parasites, as explained earlier. On the other hand, it could be sand, quartz, or flint.

It is common knowledge that a successful business needs to reduce costs to increase profits.

Food Grade Diatomaceous Earth costs anywhere from **$11** for a **10-pound bag** up to over $40 for the same size bag.

A **50-pound-bag** of sand costs **$7**.

Financially, it makes more sense to put sand in supplements.

The European Union says, "Quartz is the most common form of crystalline silica and is the second most common mineral on the earth's surface. It is found in almost every type of rock [,] i.e. [,] igneous, metamorphic and sedimentary. Since it is so abundant, quartz is present in nearly all mining operations."[ccclxiii]

The European Association of Industrial Silica Producers says, "The silica in the sand will normally be in the crystalline form of quartz. Depending on how the silica deposit was formed, quartz grains may be sharp and angular, sub-angular, sub-rounded or rounded. Foundry and filtration applications require sub-rounded or rounded grains for best performance."[ccclxiv]

Silica, a mineral, is needed in the body. It is most predominantly found in our connective tissues, skin, blood vessels, cartilage, bone, teeth, tendons, and hair. Much like a web netting, it holds us up tightly. Silica is found in high amounts in any vegetable that stands straight up like asparagus and celery, as well as in palm trees. This is silica in its natural form.

This is not sand.

You may recognize silicon dioxide from seeing it on the labels of small white rectangular packets that say "do not eat," as they absorb moisture in various products during shipping and shelf time.

The main problem with using ingredients that fill a capsule instead of food ingredients is that the body needs to process that ingredient.

Sometimes it takes a great deal of effort for the body to do this.

In his book Enzymes, *The Key to Health*, Dr. Howard Loomis says, "The body will compensate for any deviation in the contents of the blood by pulling what it needs from its tissues."[ccclxv]

He goes on to say, "Most of the vitamins and minerals that you buy at the drugstore and health food store come from the processing of wood or petroleum. Any chemist will tell you that a vitamin is a vitamin – the same molecular structure regardless of the source, natural or synthetic. The problem is science on paper does not nourish a body."[ccclxvi]

Man will never create a product as well as God himself has.

He made your body. He made the food that feeds your body. If we eat man's food, made from man's ingredients, we cannot thrive long-term. You cannot feed a body chemicals and expect it to perform in a healthy manner.

More Wood Pulp and Cotton in Your Supplements

Cellulose and microcrystalline cellulose can be found in nearly every supplement and probiotic available. Unfortunately, these items can be many things.

The International Journal of Chemical Sciences, Department of Chemical Engineering, College of Engineering and Technology in India says, "Cellulose is found in plenty in nature in the form of cotton, hemp, jute, flax etc. A good percentage of wood also consists of cellulose."[ccclxvii]

They go on to say, "Garment and hosiery industries are having the abundant waste of the cotton rags, cuttings etc. during the manufacturing of garments. As cotton is having highest percentages (87 to 96 %) of cellulose, it can be used for manufacturing of value added products like microcrystalline cellulose (MCC). Microcrystalline cellulose is very important product in pharmaceutical, food, cosmetic and other industries."[ccclxviii]

Cotton rags are not food.

Journal of Advanced Pharmaceutical Technology and Research, says, "Microcrystalline cellulose (MCCI) has been widely used as an excipient for direct compression due to its good flowability, compressibility, and compactibility. MCCI was obtained from agricultural by-products, such as corn cob, sugar cane bagasse, rice husk, and cotton by pursuing acid hydrolysis, neutralization, clarification, and drying steps."[ccclxix]

Agricultural byproducts are not food.

The Indian Journal of Pharmaceutical Sciences says, "Microcrystalline cellulose for industrial purposes is usually obtained from wood pulp and purified cotton liners. Each of these is a 'natural' source, cotton is a high value-added crop and wood pulp generally originates in some manner from deforestation."[ccclxx]

Drugs.com says, "Microcrystalline cellulose is refined wood pulp. It is a white, free-flowing powder.

Chemically, it is an inert substance, is not degraded during digestion, and has no appreciable absorption.

In large quantities, it provides dietary bulk and may lead to a laxative effect."[ccclxxi] Emphasis added.

They go on to say, "Microcrystalline cellulose is a commonly used excipient in the pharmaceutical industry. It has excellent compressibility properties and is used in solid dose forms, such as tablets. Tablets can be formed that are hard, but dissolve quickly. Microcrystalline cellulose is the same as cellulose, except that it meets USP standards."

Wood pulp and purified cotton liners are not food.

The Department of Pharmaceutical Chemistry, Faculty of Pharmacy from the University of Dhaka, the Department of Pharmacy from the State University of Bangladesh, and the Department of Pharmacy from Primeasia University put forth a report entitled "Preparation of Microcrystalline Cellulose from Cotton and its Evaluation as Direct Compressible Excipient in the Formulation of Naproxen Tablets."[ccclxxii]

When referencing microcrystalline cellulose, they say, "It is one of the mostly used filler-binders in direct tablet compression. Its popularity in direct compression is due to its excellent binding properties when used as a dry binder. In addition to its use in direct compression formulations, MCC is used as a diluent in tablets prepared by wet granulation as well as a filler for capsules and spheres."[ccclxxiii]

The purpose of their report was, of course, financial for pharmaceuticals. They said, “Traditionally, MCC has been prepared from bamboo, wood pulp, and viscose rayon. Attempts have also been made to produce MCC from other sources such as newsprint waste, corncobs, bagasse, rice straw as well as fast-growing plants.”[ccclxxiv]

Bamboo, wood pulp, and viscose rayon are not food.

Newsprint waste, corncobs, bagasse, and rice straw are not food.

If it’s not food, don’t put it in your mouth.

Soil-Based Organism Probiotics Under Attack

Bacillus subtilis, a soil-based organism contained in certain probiotics, has recently been under attack for potentially causing septicemia. Truth be told, this probiotic is not for the novice; it must be taken with knowledge of what you are doing, and it is imperative that is coincides with a proper gut healing protocol that seals any potential intestinal damage due to pathogen overgrowth. This is the case for probiotics in general, not just those containing *Bacillus subtilis*. It is always best to speak to your qualified and knowledgeable practitioner first, before beginning any protocol.

When taken properly, this exact bacterial organism is considered one of the most powerful gut healers. *B. subtilis* grows in the soil right at the level of the roots in grass or garden zones.

In 1994, the EPA saw such extreme dangers with *B. subtilis* they set forth regulation for facilities using the bacteria saying, "Standards for minimizing emission specify that liquid and solid waste containing the microorganisms be treated to give a validated decrease in viable microbial populations so that at least 99.9999 percent of the organisms resulting from the fermentation will be killed."[ccclxxv]

Like most issues regarding food today, the problem arises with the "other" form of A-amylase, as there are two. One is found naturally in food and in soil; the other is man-made.

The Food and Agriculture Organization says A-amylase "is a genetically engineered enzyme that is thermo-stable and active at a relatively low pH and low calcium concentration."[ccclxxvi]

That is why *B. subtilis* is avidly used in the production of enzymes, including commercial products, like ethanol, but is also naturally found in food. A-amylase is also the main enzyme found in humans and mammals. In addition to saliva, A-amylase is released from the pancreas, an organ that releases digestive enzymes into the intestinal tract to digest food. It is found in some seeds and mushrooms.

A-amylase is found in saliva where it breaks down starchy food. People who do not digest starchy foods have a malfunctioning breakdown occurring somewhere in their body, causing a deficiency in A-amylase. Collectively, these soil-based organism enzymes, certain chemicals, and antibiotics containing A-amylase are considered a Class 1 Containment Agent by the NIH as well as by the European Federal of Biotechnology guidelines.

The EPA goes on to say, "To date, EPA has reviewed three premanufacture notices for strains of *B. subtilis*. One of the strains was modified for enhanced production of the enzyme A-amylase to be used primarily in production of ethanol. Another strain was modified for enhanced production of a lipase enzyme for use in heavy duty detergents."[ccclxxvii] L-lipase is another enzyme that is in foods, in the body, and man-made.

The *Journal of Clinical Microbiology* says, "Data on the general importance of infections due to *B. subtilis* are incomplete, since it is a general practice of most microbiological laboratories to discard these strains or to report them as contaminants. Also, in the cause-of-death statistics of the World Health Organization no data on *B. subtilis* infections are present. *B. subtilis* spores are available in Italy as a pharmaceutical preparation for oral use. Each dose contains a mixture of 109 spores of four distinct antibiotic-resistant derivatives of ATCC 9799 (Enterogermina; distributed by Sanofi Winthrop, Milan, Italy) per vial. The pathogenic potential of *B. subtilis* is generally described as low or absent."[ccclxxviii]

They further reported (presumably) the one case in question — a 73-year-old man with recurrent septicemia resulting from chronic lymphocytic leukemia. The man showed numerous markers for Intestinal Permeability (Leaky Gut in layman's terms).[ccclxxix]

This means that whatever went into his intestinal tract also seeped into his bloodstream.

The man had been taking *B. subtilis*, reportedly, for over a month before he encountered symptoms of high fever, mental confusion, and diarrhea that caused admission to the hospital. Blood tests, in triplicate, showed *B. subtilis* in his bloodstream.

If the man had Intestinal Permeability, this would be a normal outcome of taking *B. subtilis* as the strain went directly from the intestinal tract into the bloodstream.

They administered antibiotics, the symptoms disappeared, but he remained hospitalized. *B. subtilis* was not re-administered. Sixteen days later, symptoms returned, tests again detected *B. subtilis* in his bloodstream, and more antibiotics were given. Six days later, the patient died. The *Journal of Clinical Microbiology* said, "Lymphoid cells were detected in the cerebrospinal fluid (cerebrospinal fluid was not cultured), and the patient died probably due to central nervous system involvement."[ccclxxx]

The *Journal of Neuro-Oncology* reports, "Central nervous system involvement is a rare complication of chronic lymphocytic leukemia."[ccclxxxi] This means, in some cases, that lymphocytic leukemia presents with central nervous system involvement, with or without *B. subtilis* administered orally.

Dr. Natasha McBride is a specialist in Intestinal Permeability and advocates first sealing the Intestinal Permeability.[ccclxxxii] This prevents foreign matter, including undigested food particles, putrid rotting food particles, and pathogens from leaking directly through the intestinal wall into the blood stream.

Most importantly, when you begin introducing probiotic strains that build up the good bacteria in the gut, the bad bacteria will die, releasing toxic gases and waste. Sealing the gut will mitigate these toxins from passing through into the bloodstream.

John Brisson, author of *Fix Your Gut*, has been very vocal in speaking out against *B. subtilis*, saying, "Everyone believes I have a vendetta against

HSO's (the soil-based organism *B. subtilis*). Maybe I do, maybe I do not. Honestly, I am just tired of everyone saying that HSO's or that probiotics in general have no side effects whatsoever, and that they are perfectly safe."[ccclxxxiii]

Brisson posted an article "*Bacillus Subtilis*: Any Benefit of the Bacteria Is Not Worth the Risk" where he attempts to defame *B. subtilis* but then contradicts himself, saying, "There are a few known clinical case studies that mention opportunistic *Bacillus* infections occurring in patients with compromised immune systems. One of the case reports theorizes that the main reason for such few reports of infection is that *Bacillus subtilis* is recognized by most medical professionals as a safe bacteria."[ccclxxxiv]

All gut healing includes die-off toxins that can be interpreted as ill side effects when in fact, they are signs telling the body what is happening, showing the person what to do next.

Acupuncturist and columnist for the *Huffington Post*, Chris Kresser says in an interview with Steve Wright from *SCD Lifestyle*, "Soil based organisms are a different approach than the lactic acid forming types of probiotics. I've found they're better tolerated in people with SIBO (Small Intestine Bacterial Overgrowth). As a fairly unrelated side note, they tend to work better for constipation than a lot of other probiotics. Oftentimes, probiotics can make constipation worse, so the soil-based organisms and Prescript Assist, I think, is a really good choice for people with SIBO."[ccclxxxv]

As stated, *B. subtilis* grows in the soil right at the level of the roots in grass or garden zones. Digging in the soil and not rinsing vegetables from your homegrown, non-pesticide using garden could prove beneficial. Many people sensitive to the beneficial bacteria *B. subtilis* find it necessary to cut back on dosage during the months they do garden work to keep die-off in check because they are getting *B. subtilis* naturally from working in the dirt.

Prescript Assist is quite possibly one of the most commonly taken soil-based organism probiotics, contains 29 strains of microflora from soil-based organisms, and is shelf-stable, not needing refrigeration.

The prebiotic in this probiotic has not been shown to be problematic for those with sensitive tracts.

Some people have taken vegetables right out of the garden, without washing them, and fermented them to obtain soil-based organisms in their ferments. The only complaint is that, if sand or tiny stones are in the dirt left on the vegetables, it is like eating tiny rocks in your ferment.

The Proper Way to Take Probiotics

Many people are wasting hundreds of dollars on probiotics that are not worth a dime. Knowing exactly what is happening in your body is key to healing your gut. Watching and listening to what your body is telling you is vital. Finding the strains that your body is weak in is imperative to the process. A compromised gut is made evident through illness, allergies, and even auto-immune diseases. Both over-the-counter probiotics and home-brewed probiotics are important in this process.

Your intestinal tract is a long tube, filled with a lining made up of good and bad bacteria. These bacteria alone weigh three pounds, the same weight as a brick. If you spread the tract out flat, it would cover a tennis court. When the good bacteria are killed off from antibiotics (against life), birth control pills, GMOs, pesticides, and other damaging elements, they must be rebuilt through probiotics (for life).

Probiotic foods, such as fermented coconut water, sauerkraut, kraut juice, kefir, kombucha, yogurt, kimchi, and the like, are easy to make.

The biggest challenge is your own fear.

In his book *Wild Fermentation*, Sandor Katz says there is no danger in fermenting fruits and vegetables.[ccclxxxvi] Most importantly, there has never been a report made to the FDA of a death from fermented fruit and vegetable products. During the fermentation process, there are four stages. In these stages, pathogens like *Salmonella* and botulism cannot survive, due to the specific strain formation during those stages. The two cannot live in the same environment at the same time.

Fermented fish and meats are another topic, as they are susceptible to botulism.

Ferments rank high in probiotic strains, and they give the person preparing the food the ability to introduce more strains that are specifically deficient for that person's intestinal tract. For example, fermented coconut water, a probiotic drink, is beneficial for building up the good bacteria in the gut, enabling it to fight off pathogens. Many people with yeast overgrowth say that they see powerful die-off symptoms specific to killing off yeast strains, like Candida, through fermented coconut water, sauerkraut, and kraut juice, due to the high lactobacillus content.

At the same time, some say that eating fermented foods feed yeasts and should be avoided, resulting in a dire point of confusion for many people. This point of controversy can easily be addressed through those with the most severely damaged guts, "canaries in the coalmine," who show benefits from fermented foods, even if they have pathogenic yeast strains.

When the gut is damaged at more severe levels, starting with the liquid from the ferments is protocol. If the tract cannot digest the vegetables from the ferment, they will just sit there. This stagnant, decomposing food can feed pathogens. Therefore, the greater the damage, the slower the introduction of probiotic foods must be. This situation is extremely rare. Some say that it is so rare, it is not worth discussing.

Again, while you are building the gut, it is necessary to introduce new probiotic strains, while looking for die-off: headache, runny nose, cold-like symptoms, flu-like symptoms, joint pain, body aches, anxiety, depression, confusing thoughts, sinus pain, tooth pain, diarrhea, constipation, gas, bloating, clingy behavior, laughing for no reason, bumping into walls, waking in the middle of the night, vomiting, scratchy throat, throat pain, and more. Usually die-off symptoms are specific to each person and generally follow the same pattern of symptoms caused by the illness.

For example, if your child has autism and stims with drooling, once you give him the right probiotic with strains he is weak in, his die-off symptoms may be stimming and drooling.

This is the puzzle in which Mom needs to become a detective because healing the gut is sometimes confusing for a beginner. Those with the most damaged guts may only tolerate one drop of a probiotic liquid on their tongue or one drop in a glass of water sipped throughout the day. Some need to be more extreme and put one drop in a glass of water and take one drop of that mixture per day.

This is the starting point. The biggest struggle in a situation like this is that the person feels like he or she is doing nothing and is frustrated. The point is, what the person tolerates is everything, even if it is a drop in a glass of water and taking a drop of that mixture. If that is what is tolerated, it is everything for that person.

Once the diluted drop is tolerated, after a month, people often build to two drops a day, one in the morning and one in the evening. This is increased slowly, as tolerated.

Others can drink a whole quart or two of the same probiotic liquid and not experience die-off until they drink over 2 quarts. If you can tolerate that much of those specific strains, you do not need to build those strains. Look further for other weak strains through other probiotic foods or over-the-counter strains.

Frankly, for the most part, it does not matter where you start if you start and keep building.

The goal is to look for die-off and increase the quantity, building those weak strains.

If you experience die-off, it is good. It means you are weak in these strains. You need these strains; you just do not need so much.

The Herxheimer reaction, also known as Herxing, die-off, or a healing crisis, is key to healing and recovery. This die-off reaction is your marker and tells you if you are just wasting time or building the microbiome. You want this. You are looking for this.

Some people take a fermented food, experience die-off, and say, "I have histamine issues; I can't have that."

Every situation is individual and should be evaluated for the source or cause of the situation. Often, a true histamine issue is not a situation where the mast cells are damaged; but instead, the person is experiencing die-off, or Herxing.

This is what you want; you have found the strains that your body is deficient in, and you need to focus on them, building them. When you find this weakness, go back and start slowly, building in microscopic quantities, if needed. For some, this means opening the probiotic capsule and starting with one speck or putting one drop in a teaspoon of water and taking one drop of that diluted solution. Where you start is where you start building.

It is very important that you do not remain in the stage of die-off, a status involving a lot of inflammation. The body cannot heal properly in an inflamed state.

Some people think, "Hey, let's just get a lot of die-off going on so we can get it out faster!"

This is not the case.

Once the die-off is inflaming the system, the healing mechanism stops. Again, the body cannot heal with too much probiotic, constantly Herxing.

There are certain situations in which the die-off is mild and tolerable. The person can push through in this state.

The GAPS protocol lays out the proper method for rebuilding the system through probiotic foods, probiotics, and foods that are most digestible. As the intestinal tract builds, things progress; more foods, which were not previously tolerated, can be introduced in a certain order, according to their digestibility and the killing off of pathogens.

Every person with a damaged gut will experience these die-off issues; this is merely a reflection that the weakness needs to be rebuilt. The pathogens are overgrown, but healing is occurring.

Taking the same probiotic daily is often a waste of money, especially if you have not tested your strengths in those strains. Most people in the process of healing build up to 11 capsules a day of each product, hold that dosage for a month, and then move on to other potentially weak strains, occasionally going back to the previously re-established strains to be sure they remain strong.

GAPS compliance is taking the probiotic until you reach your therapeutic dose, holding that level for six months, and then backing off slowly, while increasing a new probiotic or probiotic food.

Taking one capsule daily for years will not rebuild the gut if you are not experiencing die-off symptoms.

Histamine Issues

Histamine responses are probably the most misunderstood aspect of rebuilding the microbiome. Many people experience a reaction to a food, or certain foods, claim they have a histamine reaction, and then avoid the foods.

This is a mistake.

Full healing cannot take place with the avoidance of histamine-containing foods. Rebuilding the microbiome methodically is protocol for sealing and healing the gut.

Histamine reactions are common in people who have a compromised microbiome. The worse the damage in the gut is, the more prevalent the issue will be.

Picture a shag carpet covering a tennis court. In the shag there are balls like a child left their toys in the carpet. When the shag carpet is damaged, the balls are more like dried-up capers, leaking their air from inside when something upsets them. This is how the histidine cells release histamine.

Rebuilding the shag carpet rebuilds the balls. After a hearty protocol of GAPS meat stock, the histamine issue is resolved. From then on, die-off is the issue. For some, this takes a month or two of meat stock every hour. For others, it takes longer, but the healing still happens.

When the histidine cells release histamine, it is known to throw off the zinc and cooper balance in the body, making repair without support more difficult. If you find yourself in this situation, a good method for checking your zinc levels is with a zinc assay, a liquid zinc drink available on Amazon. Holding one teaspoon in your mouth for a few minutes will tell you right away if your zinc levels are deficient.

If the assay tastes like water, it reflects a zinc deficiency and should be swallowed as a supplement. If it tastes nasty, then spit it out; your levels fall within range.

There are several visual markers on the body that show a zinc deficiency. Collectively, they tell us the story. White spots on that nails that look like splashes of white paint can be reflective of a zinc deficiency. These spots must grow out on the nail bed to disappear. If the zinc deficiency continues, new spots will appear. Pale areas of the nail bed are also signs of a zinc deficiency. If the nails are white at the lunula, then pink, then pale, then pink, then white at the end, this is reflective of a zinc deficiency. Cracks, or splits, in the corners of the mouth, the oral commissure, are also reflective of a zinc deficiency.

Histamine issues come from a compromised microbiome. The pathogenic overload has compromised the mast cell function.

This is common and is just a reflection of the depth of damage in the gut.

The most beneficial protocol for healing histamine responses is the GAPS protocol. If you suffer from histamine issues, the protocol for the healing meat stock is to make the stock, appropriate for your body, and freeze what you will not use in two days' time.

Be sure that you are using meat stock and not bone broth.

This repair process should only take a few months.

Meat stock is high in the amino acids proline and glycine, biotin, collagen, elastin, glucosamine, and gelatin. These are the elements that feed the enterocytes, the building blocks of rebuilding the gut lining.

Feeding these amino acids feeds the histidine amino acid, rebuilding the damage.

Histidine can be replaced through protein-rich foods and by building the microflora, creating homeostasis. Kraut juice is the best way to begin building up the gut flora, as stated previously, which will help with a histamine reaction. The deeper the damage of the histidine cells is, the less kraut juice a person will be able to handle.

Science tells us that sauerkraut contains histamine. Sauerkraut comes later, after rebuilding the foundation with other probiotic foods like kvass, fermented vegetables, and kraut juice.

Starting kraut juice with a histamine sensitivity is often a slow, arduous process — so slow that it feels pathetic.

Those with the most severe damage start with kraut juice in whatever amount tolerable and build.

Many people can start their kraut juice dosage with one teaspoon of kraut juice. A person with a histamine issue cannot do this. They may start with one drop, or even with one drop in a quarter of a cup of water, taking one drop of that solution. As previously stated, some put one drop in an eight-ounce glass of water and take a drop of that, or tiny sips throughout the day.

If the amount tolerated is so low that less than one drop is taken, it is recommended that the person start by putting kraut juice into hot meat stock; this depletes the probiotic content but retains the beneficial rebuilding enzymes.

This process rebuilds what is missing in the microbiome so that repair can happen.

When we consider the interior of the intestinal tract as a long tube, cut open and covering a tennis court, we would have a shag carpet covering the tennis court with a two-inch layer of mucous on top. The balls are sporadically placed on the carpet. The shag carpet fibers are the villi with constantly surfacing enterocytes. The two-inch layer of mucous is filled with the good and bad flora.

The balls are the mast cells, hormones, and amino acids.

This is a healthy microbiome.

Comparing this to a compromised microbiome, the shag carpet is a linoleum floor. In some places there are holes in the floor. The two-inch layer of mucous is imbalanced with pathogenic overgrowth, and the mast cell "balls" are dried up and shriveled.

They are not functioning properly.

Rebuilding the whole microbiome by sealing the holes and rebuilding the good guys will feed the mast cells properly. The body repairs itself when supported properly.

Dr. Amy Myers describes histamine as "a chemical involved in your immune system, proper digestion, and your central nervous system. As a neurotransmitter, it communicates important messages from your body to your brain. It is also a component of stomach acid, which is what helps you break down food in your stomach."[cclxxxvii]

Myers is a medical doctor who practices functional medicine. She says, "Histamine causes your blood vessels to swell, or dilate, so that your white blood cells can quickly find and attack the infection or problem. If you don't break down histamine properly, you could develop what we call histamine intolerance."

In her book *The Autoimmune Solution*, she explains the process further.

Histamine is released by the body to ward off an offender; inflammation is there, acting like bubble wrap, protecting what's underneath. The job of histamine is to inflame the system, waving a flag to the immune system, screaming *Attackers are here! Fight! Fight to the death!*[cclxxxviii]

The amino acid L-histidine responds by releasing histamine. Those with illnesses such as FPIES, PANDAS, autism, schizophrenia, fibromyalgia, ME, and chronic fatigue syndrome must step lightly, progressing slowly with healing, non-inflammatory foods, rebuilding with proper probiotics, walking out of the imbalance — rebuilding.[ccclxxxix]

Again, this process can be painfully slow.

Histidine is a semi-essential amino acid that plays a part in the formation of proteins and also influences metabolic reactions. Stress, poor diet, or improper absorption of nutrients can cause nutritional deficiencies. This can deplete histidine levels; depleted levels can cause susceptibility to reactors.

Histidine transforms into histamine, glutamate, and hemoglobin, according to the body's need.

Allergies are the body's normal response; the body is doing what it is designed to do – to create an inflammatory response as protection from the offender. This inflammation is sourced from the mast cells and basophils (white blood cells), which both contain histamine.

When a person is dehydrated the process is exacerbated. This means that if you are dehydrated, you may experience heightened histamine issues.

Water Cures says that, with dehydration, "your histamine levels are elevated. This results in suppressed white blood cell production, the very things that help you eliminate allergy responses."[cccxc]

When the body is dehydrated it will release more histamine as a method of guarding the body to prevent further dehydration.[cccxci]

The histamine issue is not a simple process, because it functions on different levels from different sources and can even enter your system on food that has been cooked for too long or is not fresh. Eating food that has been in the refrigerator for too long can cause what is referred to as a histamine reaction; however, this area is up for debate among professionals.

Some say that it is not necessarily a histamine reaction, but instead, a response to the pathogens growing on the food, which cause reactions in a hypersensitive tract, due to an imbalance in the microbiome.

The older the food is, the less nutrition it contains. Cooked food grows pathogens with age. This is not necessarily a histamine reaction, but it is a reaction to the pathogens growing on older food.

Amino Acid Studies says, "Histidine regulates the immune defense in the body, allergic reactions and inflammatory processes, so a deficiency of L-histidine can lead to an increased tendency towards infection and the aggravation of symptoms of allergies."[cccxcii]

Histidine is known to be ambiguous. It prefers a comfortable, secure location, like burrowed deep in a protein core. It also functions as a solvent out and about in the body. The body releases histamine to do exactly that — to work as a solvent against offenders. When the solvent is released, and the bubble wrap coating is in place, the body is doing its job. However, when there is too much, and the body is in overdrive, more is released than the body can handle – this is an allergic reaction. This histamine response comes in the form of itchy eyes, runny nose, cold symptoms, flu symptoms, tightness in the chest, hives, rash, stomach upset, gas, and bloating, as well as others.[cccxciii]

Histamine reactions are the same types of responses that a person gets from the die-off of pathogens. In fact, a great deal of what is thought to be histamine issues is simply die-off.

Dr. Natasha teaches all Certified GAPS Practitioners in Training, "I wouldn't focus on histamine too much. It is die-off."[cccxciv]

It is important to remember that these pathogens are living beings. When they are thriving, they are exhaling, pooping, peeing, burping, and releasing their toxic gases.

When we feed the good through probiotic food, it fights the bad; the bad dies, releasing all of its toxic gases.

Determining which is happening to your body can be done by you.

Histamine responses will follow food; die-off will follow probiotics or probiotic foods. Some foods give die-off responses but carry histamine, causing confusion.

Kraut juice and sauerkraut follow this pattern and are the biggest offenders for most people.

This is a good sign and is evidence that you need these strains of probiotics. Again, you are weak in these strains; you just don't need so much.

It does not mean that you should drop them.

If you experience this, follow the proper introductory stage for probiotics, beginning with kraut juice fermented for 12 days, or much longer, with the cabbage pieces fully submerged under the brine. The quantity you can handle is specific to your pathogen overload, and no one can tell you what to start with; only your body can do that.

If the tolerated kraut juice is in the one drop range, it is important to rebuild other probiotics at the same time, such as with dairy introduction, kvass, and others.

Stopping sauerkraut juice because it gives you a reaction will only prolong the pathogen overgrowth. Building slowly — very, very, slowly — ideally, with the guidance of a skilled practitioner knowledgeable in this area, can be important to healing. Histamine can be put in check with proper rebuilding.

Amino Acid Studies adds, "Once formed, histamine is either stored or broken down by an enzyme. Histamine in the central nervous system is broken down primarily by histamine N-methyltransferase (HMT), while histamine in the digestive tract is broken down primarily by diamine oxidase (DAO).

Both enzymes play an important role in histamine break down."[cccxcv]

The American Society for Clinical Nutrition says that the enzyme DAO breaks down histamine introduced through the mouth, in food. Eating foods that are not fresh will create a histamine response in those with great intestinal damage. For this reason, while healing the body of the histamine response, it is vital to eat fresh food and fresh meat stock.[cccxcvi]

Allergies begin in the gut from a damaged microbiome. Sealing and healing the gut with meat stock, while building up the good bacteria, prevents the reaction and cycle of histamine, halting the allergen response at the source.

The homeopathy remedy histaminum is designed to stop a histamine reaction. Most importantly, there are no adverse effects known from homeopathy, and it will not cause drowsiness like over-the-counter antihistamine products, even for an infant, pet, or elderly person. Histaminum is recommended for any antihistamine needs, where histamines are an issue, including sneezing, watery eyes, congestion, itching, hives, food allergies, and burning eyes or throat, due to allergens.

This homeopathic antihistamine is reported safe for any age by homeopaths. Proper protocol for homeopathy is 4 tablets under the tongue. If symptoms remain 15 minutes later, repeat the dosage.

Repeat again 15 minutes later if needed; back off as needed.

Be cautious, as some people experience wheezing if they take histaminum hydrochloricum with belladonna.

Homeopathy: The Journal of the Faculty of Homeopathy reported a study on homeopathic histaminum and cat saliva in regard to cat allergies. They tested 30 individuals who tested positive to a cat allergy on the skin prick test (SPT) through a double-blind, randomized, placebo-controlled study.[cccxcvii]

They reported, "Cat saliva 9cH and Histaminum 9cH produced a highly statistically significant reduction in the wheal diameter of the cat allergen SPT at the end of week 4. The placebo group showed no statistically significant change. The homeopathic medicine reduced the sensitivity reaction of cat allergic adults to cat allergen, according to the SPT."[cccxcviii]

Rescue Remedy, a Bach Flower remedy, also stops histamine reactions naturally. It is much quicker at stopping a die-off reaction, but it does work for both.

If you are experiencing histamine responses, it is a sign that you have great intestinal imbalance in your microflora. This is good news, as there is a specific protocol for healing this issue laid out in the GAPS book. Those with histamine issues are the easiest to heal because their bodies speak to them throughout the healing process, telling them what to and what not to do. It often takes longer for healing to occur, however, especially with age.

Many histamine responses come from bones and meats from animals fed GMO feed or animal products that have been injected with preservatives or flavorings or have been sprayed with bleach for sanitation. If you experience this situation, source cleaner animals. The easiest way to do this is to contact friends who are hunters and ask them for the bones from their kill. The best option in this case is to bake cookies for the man in your area who processes deer and other animals for hunters. He can be found with a simple Google search of your area. He is most likely throwing the valuable bones away. If the reaction mentioned above occurs, it is not a histamine issue; it is a pathogen issue.

The repair of a histamine issue for the person who suffering from histamine responses is similar to the old dog on a nail scenario. Imagine you see an old dog, moaning while curled into a pile on the floor. He moans and moans and moans, and yet does nothing. You ask, "Why is he moaning?" It is because he is lying on a nail. "Why doesn't he move?" It is because it doesn't hurt him badly enough.

If people are hurting enough, they will generally act on rebuilding. If not, they may just avoid their problem areas, eliminating food after food after food, until their food choices are pitifully limited. It is important to remember that avoiding problem areas often results in further decline of the ecosystem from where the problem is sourced.

Folks who respond to bone broth with a histamine response are hurt badly enough to do something about it. This is an advantage. Those who are not hurting enough have no real motivation to change their ways, so they often do not. Then they slowly, but surely, get more and more ill over the course of time, while the histamine person gets better because they are sick and tired of being sick and tired.

Bone broth is not recommended for those with a histamine issue because it is cooked too long. Meat stock is the solution that is recommended.

Die-off and histamine issues are encountered by most people while attempting to repair the damage. However, when you progress in a certain rhythm, according to Dr. Natasha's protocol, histamines are not an issue.

A histamine or die-off response is your body talking to you, telling you what is happening in the gut. It is a good sign. Probiotic foods are the very thing that your body needs in order to heal and to rebuild the good flora in the intestinal tract.

Histamines can accumulate in your body and then result in an explosive reaction, often through a raised red rash that resembles a burn. Histamine responses can be flushing of the face and body, nausea, burning in the mouth, headache, feeling faint, blurred vision, abdominal cramps, gas, diarrhea, wheezing, respiratory issues, cold-like symptoms, flu-like symptoms, swelling or inflammation, hives, eczema, or other similar responses.

When dealing with GAPS, the intestinal tract is loaded with pathogenic bacteria, which is killed off by probiotic foods and capsules. Die-off symptoms are a raised red rash that resembles a burn, flushing of the face and body, nausea, burning in the mouth, headache, feeling faint, blurred vision, abdominal cramps, gas, diarrhea, wheezing, respiratory issues, cold-like symptoms, flu-like symptoms, swelling or inflammation, hives, eczema, acne, marks that look like red ant bites, exhaustion, irritation, anger, and a short temper.

Notice the similarity in symptoms between die-off and histamine issues. This causes confusion for many people.

Often, people with histamine issues remove probiotic healing foods to avoid the histamine reaction. When histamine issues are evident, it is vital to go back a step and begin healing with gentler probiotic foods like unpasteurized whey (as part of the dairy introduction) and kraut juice, giving the intestinal tract time to heal.

Dr. Judy Tsafrir, MD says, "FODMAPS and Histamine Intolerance are not primary conditions, but rather secondary manifestations which have resulted from gut inflammation and damage via dysbiosis."[cccxcix]

Most probiotics purchased in the store are filled with ingredients not conducive to gut healing; instead, they feed bad bacteria in the gut, making matters worse.

The only way to know how much probiotic your body should take is to try some and see how your body responds. If the symptoms are reflective of deeper damage, having Rescue Remedy nearby, as previously stated, is best.

People who have mild gut damage can tolerate larger doses of fermented foods. It is more beneficial to take smaller amounts of probiotic foods throughout the day, rather than to take one large dose and encounter a great deal of die-off. Kraut juice and whey are both good introductory probiotic foods for damaged guts, especially for those that experience these symptoms.

If you suffer from too much die-off, going back even further to fermented cucumbers (called probiotic pickles), fermented green beans, fermented asparagus, and home-brewed whey, is protocol.

On page 29 of GAPS FAQs (Frequently Asked Questions) Dr. Natasha clearly answers the histamine issue:

Q: Is the GAPS Diet appropriate for someone with histamine intolerance?[cd]

A: Yes! I believe that people with this condition have an overgrowth of particular species of microbes in the gut which produce histamine and block the enzyme (diamine oxidase), which is supposed to process histamine. GAPS Program will allow you to change your gut flora and remove this condition permanently. In the initial stages avoid all the culprit foods: all alcohol, black tea, canned and smoked foods, leftovers (you should eat everything as fresh as possible), beans and lentils, fermented vegetables, mature cheeses, cocoa, nuts, etc. All fresh foods prepared at home, including freshly fermented yogurt and kefir will be fine for you. It will be best if you follow the GAPS Introduction Diet.[cdi]

On page 14 of GAPS FAQs, she goes into a deeper explanation.[cdii]

Q: Your book has a single chapter on sauerkraut saying it is ready in 5-7 days, but other research has shown that in the first 2-3 weeks histamines are released which can cause major reactions which are not a problem at the end of a longer 6 weeks fermentation process. Does fermenting vegetables longer decrease the histamine levels in the food.[cdiii]

A: In the majority of my patients following the recipe in my book works. For people who are particularly sensitive to histamines it may make sense to ferment their vegetables longer.[cdiv]

On page 19 of FAQs:

Q: How long will it take to heal histamine intolerance and how long will it take before fermented veggies can be introduced? Are there any specific supplements you suggest to help with this intolerance?[cdv]

A: It is very individual how long it takes to heal. Keep testing if you are getting more tolerant by trying to eat tomato, eggplant or spinach before trying to eat fermented vegetables. I believe that it is the abnormal flora that produces excessive amounts of histamine and also impairs enzymes which break the histamine down in the body.[cdvi]

Patricia Allen, Certified Nutritional Therapist and Certified GAPS Practitioner in Atlanta says, "The pathogenic microbes continually produce toxins from their life cycle. They flood the brain with toxins and can cause people to feel drunk. They produce a group of substances called amines and produce too much histamines."[cdvii]

Allen goes on to say, "Some amines produced by pathogenic microbes from amino acids like choline, lecithin, methylamine, lysine, arginine, ornithine, and tyrosine have been shown to cause intellectual regression, behavior and emotional issues, and withdrawal symptoms."[cdviii]

When these amines are circulating through the bloodstream, traveling from the intestinal tract to the brain through the vagus nerve, it can produce erratic behaviors. This whole cycle needs to be stopped for recovery to happen.

Stopping Die-Off Dead in Its Tracks

Experiencing die-off is a normal part of balancing the microbiome; finding yourself in a healing crisis is a different, potentially painful, and debilitating story.

When you feed the good bacteria in your gut, it kills the bad pathogens. When they die, they release toxic gases, which can make you very ill.

Pulling yourself out of a healing crisis is simple and should not be feared.

When you find yourself in a healing crisis, there are tools in the toolbox you can use to pull yourself out of the situation quickly and naturally.

As stated earlier, Rescue Remedy is a Bach Flower Remedy that ranks number one for halting a healing crisis. Rescue Remedy is a combination of five different Bach Flowers including Impatiens, Star of Bethlehem, Cherry Plum, Rock Rose, and Clematis. It can be used in a crisis when the proper Bach Flower is not available or if the proper remedy is unknown. It is highly effective.

One dose consists of four drops under the tongue, repeating every 15 minutes until symptoms subside. Normal dosage patterns for many extreme cases follow this type of pattern: take a dose; 15 minutes later, take a dose; 15 minutes later, take a dose; 30 minutes later, take a dose; 45 minutes later, take a dose; 1 hour and 15 minutes later, take a dose; 2 hours later, take a dose; etc. Once the symptoms are gone, the remedy has done its job. If they return, another dose is protocol. This scenario is an example.

Only your body can tell you what it needs.

The drops of Rescue Remedy need to absorb into your blood stream through the mucus membranes; therefore, the remedy is dropped under the tongue. If swallowed, the remedy is not effective, as it is negated by the hydrochloric acid in your stomach. Dr. Edward Bach says that the only reasons a remedy does not work appropriately is because you are not taking enough of it, you are not taking it frequently enough, or it is the wrong remedy. Rescue Remedy is the specific remedy for die-off or a healing crisis.

Be aware, not all forms of Rescue Remedy are beneficial to healing. One variation comes in the form of pastilles that contain sugar alcohols as well as other ingredients that feed pathogens in the gut, making your issue worse in the long run. Another form assists with sleep; however, it contains sorbitol, a sugar alcohol, which feeds gut pathogens.

Drinking hot herbal tea will also assist in a healing crisis. Be sure to use loose leaf herbal teas like mint, chamomile, nettles, or the like. Making tea out of freshly grated ginger is also beneficial, as it is a prokinetic. The standard measure for tea, in this form, is one teaspoon of dried herb or ginger to one cup of water, preferably steeped for 10 to 15 minutes.

Chamomile tea is specifically known for pulling toxins out through the urine. This can be evidenced by not feeling the need to urinate but then getting the feeling to urinate immediately. This generally happens due to the toxins overburdening the bladder so that the bladder contracts immediately, trying to eliminate the toxic liquid — the same way vomiting is the stomach getting rid of toxins immediately.

Using loose leaf tea ensures that you do not feed pathogens with free-flowing agents, natural flavors, or any other pathogen-feeding ingredients commonly added to tea bags.

Another way to remedy a healing crisis is to do a detox bath. Taking detox baths every day opens the detox pathways through the skin, the largest organ of the body. Detox baths should consist of a half to one cup of Epsom salt, mineral salts, apple cider vinegar, bentonite clay, baking soda, or sea weed on a rotation cycle. Many people lean toward Epsom salt one night, mineral salts the next night, then Epsom salt, then apple cider vinegar, then Epsom salt, then baking soda, then Epsom salt, then sea weed, then Epsom salt, and then repeating the whole cycle. Only your body can tell you what to use for your detox bath. The more toxic your body is, the less you will tolerate; you will need a lower measure of salts, vinegar, etc.

Taking a detox bath during a healing crisis will help pull out some of the toxins that the body is trying to eradicate.

Meat stock is another way of assisting the body through a healing crisis.

Keeping die-off levels at a level that is barely noticeable is safe, whereas pushing the levels can cause damage.

Psychology Today reported, "As far back as 1929 it was discovered that human carriers of certain *Clostridium* species who were given epinephrine to treat hives died suddenly of gas gangrene. For 60 years, it was thought the epinephrine somehow suppressed the immune system, leading to the sudden fulminant infection. In the early 1990s, however, it was found that yes, indeed, gut bacteria could respond directly to human neurochemicals (such as epinephrine)."[cdix]

The declined ecosystem in the microbiome shows an abundance of pathogens. Something caused the good guys to die, and the bad guys bloomed, taking over the space. When pathogens bloom, it causes more pathogens to keep the balance. It is natural and normal.

The deeper the damage is, the more specific the repair must be, because the overload of toxic gases are rampant. This is the situation where going slowly, feeding the good, is vital. Going too quickly will cause too many toxic gases. In situations like this, S L O W is your friend.

The Proper Protocol for Taking Probiotics While Taking Antibiotics

Antibiotics are in our meats, our vegetables, our fruits, and our milk — not just in our medication.[cdx] [cdxi] [cdxii] [cdxiii]

Antibiotics are even in our water supply, along with other medications like antidepressants, mood stabilizers, birth control, hormones, and other medicines.[cdxiv] The function of antibiotics is to kill bacteria. However, antibiotics are indiscriminate and kill our beneficial flora, as they kill the pathogenic flora. In fact, decreased flora counts are being passed down from generation to generation, with each subsequent age having less diversity and more allergies, autism, and autoimmunity.

"The more the diversity, the happier we will be. The less the diversity, the more we've killed off; the less the diversity, the more trouble we will get from it," says Dr. Natasha Campbell-McBride.[cdxv]

Rebuilding the flora decreased by antibiotic use is vital. However, the question is presented frequently, "Do I take probiotics while I'm on antibiotics when the antibiotics are just going to kill the good bacteria anyway?"

Dr. McBride says, when it comes to administering probiotics while on antibiotics, "Start it right from the beginning. Continue taking it through the antibiotic period — just not in the same mouthful — at different times during the day."[cdxvi]

Repopulating the microbiome should not come just from capsules; it should come from food. Dr. McBride says, "Eat plenty of fermented foods. Drink kefir; eat yogurt; eat sauerkraut; make your fermented salads; make kvass."[cdxvii]

She goes on to say, "When the course of antibiotics is finished, continue taking the probiotics and eat a GAPS introduction diet. If you eat only [chicken meat stock] for a couple of days along with kefir and yogurt, your gut flora will restore itself."[cdxviii]

These foods are very soothing, anti-inflammatory, and nutritious for the digestive system.

Natural Antibiotics That Work

Thankfully, there are many natural alternatives that show quantitative results without damaging the good bacteria or causing ill effects. Taking prescribed antibiotics should be a last-ditch effort to cure disease. Using antibiotics prolifically has been shown to cause increased health challenges in the long run.

These are just a handful of the natural remedies for antibiotic use.

Propolis, made by bees from tree resin, "offers the same immediate action as laboratory produced antibiotics, but without toxic or other side effects," says Ray Hill[cdxix] in his book *Propolis – The Natural Antibiotic*. The resin is naturally anti-microbial and anti-viral, as it is what protects the tree.

In his book *The Male Herbal, Herbalist,* James Green says, "Propolis contains a complex of biologically active enzymes, vitamins, minerals and a special combination of flavonoids which act as cell building components."[cdxx]

Green recommends taking propolis straight or making an extract from it.

He goes on to say, "These properties work to raise the body's natural resistance to disease by stimulating and rejuvenating the body's own immune system. The saliva becomes activated by the resins, and as the saliva is continually swallowed, it efficiently distributes the anti-microbial components of the propolis throughout the throat and adjacent areas."[cdxxi]

If the saliva begins to sting your mouth, due to the properties which make it so beneficial, remove the propolis for ten minutes; then, repeat as tolerated.

Propolis is made by the bees collecting the resin, re-metabolizing it while commingling bee secretions, and producing a glue-like substance. The bees use this glue for hive repairs. They also use it to clean the hive, as a disinfectant. It is strategically placed at the entrance to their hives as well as around any intruding insects that the bees have killed.

Chewing propolis should be done with care, because it is quite sticky. Sucking on it for some time first, and then kneading it with your tongue against the palate is easier to manage without it sticking to your teeth. Chewing the product later, after you have worked it a bit, causes less adhesion to the teeth. Some propolis is stickier than others, depending on the resin from the specific tree that the bees used for harvesting.

Colloidal silver is another natural antibiotic; however, it should be used with caution, as it is still a heavy metal which will not be eliminated from the body, even with proactive chelation therapy. Silver does not leave the body; it just accumulates. Overuse of colloidal silver has been shown to turn people blue. As a heavy metal, silver will not assist in the long run with eliminating yeast; it will only prolong the suffering, as Candida albicans surround heavy metals inside the body to protect the body from the metal toxicity. The yeast will not leave until the metals have been eliminated.

Web MD says, "Colloidal silver is a mineral. Despite promoters' claims, silver has no known function in the body and is not an essential mineral supplement. Colloidal silver products were once available as over-the-counter products, but in 1997, the U.S. Food and Drug Administration (FDA) ruled that colloidal silver drug products were not considered safe or effective. Colloidal silver products marketed for medical purposes or promoted for unproven uses are now considered 'misbranded' under the law."[cdxxii]

However, WebMD goes on to say, "Colloidal silver can kill certain germs by binding to and destroying proteins." Silver showed great success when used in infections due to yeast, multiple forms of bacteria, tuberculosis, Lyme disease, bubonic plague, pneumonia, leprosy, gonorrhea, syphilis, scarlet fever, stomach ulcers, cholera, parasites, ringworm, malaria, and viruses such as HIV/AIDS, pneumonia, herpes, shingles, and warts.

WebMD continues to explain the benefits of colloidal silver by saying that it is used for lung conditions (including emphysema and bronchitis), skin conditions (including rosacea, cradle cap, also known as atopic dermatitis, eczema, impetigo, and psoriasis), as well as inflammation (sometimes due to infection of the bladder, prostate, colon, nose, stomach, tonsils, appendix, and sinuses), cancer, diabetes, arthritis, lupus, chronic fatigue syndrome, leukemia, hay fever and other allergies, trench foot, and gum disease, flu, H1N1 (known as swine flu), and the common cold.[cdxxiii]

Some people make their own colloidal silver, which is cheaper, however, unregulated. This practice is ill-advised; many professionals consider the molecules to be too large, leading to a greater potential of the skin turning blue. With overuse, if the person turns blue, the blue color will fill the mucous membranes, meaning that the skin will be blue, the whites of the eyes will be blue, inside the nose and ears will be blue, etc.

Garlic was nicknamed Russian Penicillin during World War II, after the country ran dry on antibiotics.

It is a powerhouse when it comes to natural antibiotic properties.

The NYU Langone Medical Center says, "Raw garlic can kill a wide variety of microorganisms by direct contact, including fungi, bacteria, viruses, and protozoa. A double-blind study reported in 1999 found that a cream made from the garlic constituent ajoene was just as effective for fungal skin infections as the standard drug terbinafine. These findings may explain why garlic was traditionally applied directly to wounds in order to prevent infection (but keep in mind that it can burn the skin)."[cdxxiv]

No scientific double-blind study shows remarkable evidence of garlic working internally. For this reason, it is considered by most medical scientists to be an antiseptic, not an antibiotic. This makes sense because it costs money to do double-blind studies, and pharmaceutical companies are often behind the funding of double-blind studies.

Many people say that garlic is the victor when it comes to easing their suffering from *Candida* overgrowth. This can be done by adding garlic to green juices, freshly pressed with a juicer. It can also be done through fermentation of garlic.

Manuka honey, a product of New Zealand, has proven to be effective in the same manner, killing pathogens.

Asian Pacific Journal of Tropical Biomedicine says, "Honey is an ancient remedy for the treatment of infected wounds, which has recently been 'rediscovered' by the medical profession, particularly where conventional modern therapeutic agents fail."[cdxxv] They go on to say that the antimicrobial agents assist in the healing of ulcers, bed sores, and skin infections.

"Many researchers have reported the antibacterial activity of honey and found that natural unheated honey has some broad-spectrum antibacterial activity when tested against pathogenic bacteria, oral bacteria as well as food spoilage bacteria," they say.[cdxxvi]

Can Probiotics Create Ethanol in Your Body?

"As you introduce probiotic bacteria in a digestive system, they start destroying pathogenic bacteria, viruses and fungi. When these pathogens die they release toxins,"[cdxxvii] says Dr. Natasha.

McBride goes on to say, "These are the toxins which made your patient autistic or schizophrenic or hyperactive."[cdxxviii]

Her studies of autism, ADHD, schizophrenia, dyslexia, dyspraxia, and other psychological problems led her to ethanol and acetaldehyde gases within the body.

Overgrowth of pathogenic flora, specifically yeasts in the *Candida albicans* family, create a revolving door within the tract.

She says, "In healthy people dietary glucose gets converted into lactic acid, water and energy through a biochemical process called glycolysis. In people with yeast overgrowth, Candida hijacks the glucose and digests it in a different way, called alcoholic fermentation. In this biochemical process Candida and other yeasts convert dietary glucose into alcohol (ethanol) and its by-product acetaldehyde."[cdxxix]

PubChem, An Open Chemistry Database says, "Ethanol is a clear, colorless liquid rapidly absorbed from the gastrointestinal tract and distributed throughout the body. It has bactericidal activity and is used often as a topical disinfectant. It is widely used as a solvent and preservative in pharmaceutical preparations."[cdxxx]

They go on to say that ethanol vapors are heavier than air. They also say that ethanol has a burning taste when in the mouth. Ethanol and the by-products of ethanol have very small molecules, allowing them to readily cross barriers within the body.[cdxxxi]

McBride says, "They get absorbed into the blood very quickly and have a very good ability to get through the placenta to a developing fetus. Overgrowing yeast in a pregnant woman would produce alcohol and its by-products, affecting the child's development."[cdxxxii]

Some say that this is one of the reasons certain women feel so good while pregnant — there is a continual stream of alcohol in their bloodstream.

"There is no part of the body that will not suffer from the constant supply of alcohol even in tiny amounts," McBride says.[cdxxxiii] She goes on to say that it directly effects reduction of stomach acid, reduction of pancreatic enzymes impairing digestion, damage to the microbiome, nutritional deficiencies (specifically vitamins A and B), decreased immune function, liver damage, brain damage, peripheral nerve damage resulting in muscle weakness, and direct muscle tissue damage.

Ethanol is directly linked to fatty liver disease.

The Cleveland Clinic says, "Nonalcoholic fatty liver disease (NAFLD) is one of the most common causes of chronic liver disease. It is strongly associated with obesity and insulin resistance and is currently considered by many as the hepatic component of the metabolic syndrome."[cdxxxiv] This is a direct result of ethanol, alcohol.

One study of test rats showed that when they were fed a liquid ethanol diet, their glutathione levels plummeted.[cdxxxv]

Proceedings of the National Academy of Sciences reported the study substituting ethanol for sucrose. They said, "The liquid ethanol diet contained 30% ethanol-derived calories. Mice were fed the indicated diets for 11–14 days and euthanized, and spleens or lymph nodes were removed aseptically for use in culture. Mice show markedly diminished delayed hypersensitivity (DTH, a Th1-associated response) and enhanced humoral immune (Th2-associated) responses. Similarly, ethanol feeding decreases OVA-specific DTH in unimmunized αβ T cell receptor transgenic (DO11.10) mice."

This creates a spiraling down effect in which the study concluded, "Our findings suggest that alteration in immune function because glutathione depletion in antigen-presenting cell populations may play a key role in exacerbating HIV and other infectious diseases in which Th2 predominance is an important aspect of the disease pathology."[cdxxxvi]

When fed ethanol, the gut flora is directly impacted, creating a deeper imbalance in the good/bad strains.

Another test study on mice fed 5% alcohol showed this decline. The journal *PLOS One* reported the study, saying, "Chronic ethanol feeding caused a decline in the abundance of both Bacteriodetes and Firmicutes phyla, with a proportional increase in the gram negative Proteobacteria and gram positive Actinobacteria phyla; the bacterial genera that showed the biggest expansion were the gram negative alkaline tolerant Alcaligenes and gram positive Corynebacterium."[cdxxxvii]

An imbalance of Bacteriodetes and Firmicutes phyla is directly associated with obesity.

They go on to say, "Tight junction (TJ) proteins play a critical role in maintaining the gut barrier integrity and can be affected by ethanol exposure leading to gut barrier dysfunction and an increase in intestinal permeability. Chronic ethanol exposure disrupts TJ proteins."[cdxxxviii]

Ethanol off-gassing is often found in people who respond in a drunk manner after a high carbohydrate meal. "Carbohydrates are consumed by Candida with the production of alcohol. Despite the fact that these people did not consume alcohol, they developed some typical symptoms of alcoholism," McBride says.[cdxxxix]

Her protocol emphasizes drowning out the pathogenic bacteria with beneficial bacteria while reducing inflammatory food intake. Probiotics are the best way to drown out the pathogens. Too much probiotic intake causes too many pathogens to die, releasing their toxic gases all at once, causing the flood of ethanol.

Each pathogen releases different toxic gases. Too many of these pathogens dying at one time, in a position where too many toxic gases are trapped in the body, can cause several symptoms, such as bloating, joint pain, headaches, diarrhea, constipation and vomiting, among others.

Too much die-off over an extended period of time causes these toxic gases to remain in certain areas of the body, which can cause extensive damage.

Taking probiotics properly is vital to recovery, for this reason.

Reading Your Stool to Decipher Your Probiotics

Many naturopathic doctors say, "Follow the poop!" Sounds like a crappy idea, but it works.

In fact, a good portion of our elimination processes are filled with pathogenic bacteria, not just with the food and drink we consume.

"All bacteria multiply very quickly. They produce trillions of babies in the blink of an eye. They don't live very long. They die. [Feces are] their dead bodies plus the organic matter that they live on in the bowel," says McBride.[cdxl]

The fecal matter is made up of bacteria, the organic matter they live on, toxic substances and by-products from our metabolism as they are eliminated from all organs and muscles, as well as food that is passing through.

"Many things inside the body will alter our beneficial flora. All pharmaceutical drugs taken on a regular basis will do that. Contraceptive[s] alter the gut flora and the whole flora quite substantially. It has a devastating effect," McBride says.[cdxli]

The Bristol Stool Chart describes texture and shape; optimal results rank right in the middle of the chart.

Color and frequency are telling.

Color is directly changed with alterations of bilirubin content. Bilirubin is a breakdown product of blood.

Medicine says, "The presence of the bilirubin in bile is generally responsible for stool color. Bilirubin concentration can vary the color of bile color from light yellow to almost black in color. Changes in bilirubin can cause stool to turn green, gray, or clay-like in color. Intestinal bleeding may turn stool black, tarry, red, maroon, or smelly. Medication and food may also affect stool color."[cdxlii]

WebMD says, "Bleeding that happens higher up in the digestive tract may make stool appear black and tarry."[cdxliii]

Bleeding in the lower region of the tract would appear more as wet, bright, red blood.

Red or dark stool is most often associated with eating beets. Green is often connected to eating certain vegetables but can also have other sources.

Continual blood in the stool is generally related to irritable bowel related inflammation and irritation. This happens when the microbiome is greatly damaged and cannot process fiber. Raw vegetables, in situations as discussed previously, can be very damaging because they irritate the inflammation further.

The Mayo Clinic says, "All shades of brown and even green are considered normal. Only rarely does stool color indicate a potentially serious intestinal condition."[cdxliv]

They go on to say, "Food may be moving through the large intestine too quickly, such as due to diarrhea. As a result, bile doesn't have time to break down completely."[cdxlv]

Bile is generally the marker for stool color and concern. Tan, gray, or white colored stool is an indicator that the bile ducts may be clogged. This can be the result of parasites, stones, or adverse responses to medications.

Metallic green is generally indicative of a specific breed of parasites.

Yellow or greasy looking stool is generally related to the fat content of the stool. If the person is eating plenty of healthy fats such as avocado, unrefined coconut oil, grass-fed butter, and pastured animal fats, and the stool has this effect, is fuzzy in appearance, and floats, it could mean that there is malabsorption, due to an altered microbiome.

Supporting the body, as previously discussed, allows the body to repair this on its own. When you support the body, according to what it needs, it can repair itself.

Fuzzy, independent circles within the stool itself could indicate parasites.

Mucus in the stool is the bowel's way of cleaning itself. Mucus in the stool works in much of the same way as mucus in the nasal cavity, lifting out offending pollen, dander, germs, etc. If parasites, worms, or bacteria are being eliminated, mucus will often be present, lubricating the pathway out of the tract.

It can work both ways, however. If we feed the pathogens, the mucus will proliferate, trying to remove the toxic overload. If we are not feeding the pathogens, the body is cleaning itself.

Gastroenterologist, Dr. Michael Samach says that it is probably nothing to worry about; "mucus is made normally as a lubricant and sometimes especially if patients are a bit constipated or straining they can see it in the stool."[cdxlvi]

By far, mucus in the stool is something that scares people the most, when in fact, if the person is eating a healing and rebuilding diet, it is an optimal sign. It shows that the body is flushing out toxins, parasites, and yeasts.

Many people add in inflammation-reducing foods and/or probiotic foods and see worms, yeast, and mucus pass through with their stool. When you build the body up, you make it stronger. A strong body can fight the pathogens all on its own.

Candida, an opportunistic yeast in the stool, has a wide variety of appearances. It is one of hundreds of yeast varieties that live in the body. It can range from a mucous-white appearance, to a snotty-looking, stringy or clumping yellow appearance, to a solid, white, spongy appearance, much like an o.b. tampon. It most commonly looks like a tissue, blown into tiny particles.

The Mycosis, a journal that covers diagnosis, therapy, and prophylaxis of fungal diseases, reported a study of Candida-positive test subjects, saying that they contained "Candida-vaginitis, allergies against food and allergies in general."[cdxlvii]

Items in the stool that look like seeds might be anything from ingested seeds passing through to eggs or segments of parasites or worms. Some worms exist one at a time but lay thousands of eggs daily.

A fecal stone is a firm ball of fecal matter filled with parasite eggs. This looks like a poo-ball filled with seeds.

Yellow to tan in color, gelatinous formations may be biofilm colonies.

All of these things can be instigated or eradicated through food. They exist for a reason, doing what the body is supposed to do by perfect design.

If probiotic foods are added to the diet, die-off and changes in the stool are normal. As the body rebuilds itself, it will eliminate pathogens. Some come out through the skin, some through the urine, and most through the bowel. A general rule of thumb is to eat clean and monitor the stools. Loose stools, hard stools, colored stools — they all mean something, telling you what to do.

Newborns and Probiotics

Newborns today are experiencing illness, rashes, digestive issues, and food intolerances more than any generation before them. Today, it is common for a toddler or child to have food allergies, eczema, constipation, or diarrhea. Rebuilding the microbiome for these children is not just about adding in healthy strains; it is about training the bacteria how to function.

The beneficial bacteria in the microbiome can be trained how to regenerate, communicate, and function properly.

"Establishment of normal gut flora in the first 20, or so, days of life plays a crucial role in appropriate maturation of the baby's immune system. Babies who develop abnormal gut flora are left immune compromised," says McBride.[cdxlviii]

Babies, overall, do not have the clean start in life that they used to have.

Scientific American reported, "The Environmental Working Group's study commissioned five laboratories to examine the umbilical cord blood of 10 babies of African-American, Hispanic and Asian heritage and found more than 200 chemicals in each newborn."[cdxlix]

WebMD says, "Infants given probiotics during the first three months of life appear to have fewer bouts of colic, acid reflux and constipation, according to Italian researchers."[cdl]

Donna Gates says, "In the first critical days after birth, one of the most important steps you can take that will determine the health and long-term wellness of your baby will be to ensure the proper development and maintenance of her *inner ecosystem*. Because 80% of the immune system is located in the gut associated lymphoid tissue (GALT), babies who do not quickly develop a healthy inner ecosystem in their gut have weakened immunity. They are also more vulnerable to allergies and other more serious problems, including autism."[cdli]

Gates further says, "Giving your baby beneficial bacteria soon after birth can ensure proper colonization of healthy microflora in their intestines and prevent food allergies that are so common today."[cdlii]

Healthline News says, "Giving infants a probiotic during their first three months of life can help prevent stomach problems like colic."[cdliii]

JAMA Pediatrics says, "Of the 12 trials (1,825 infants) reviewed, 6 suggested probiotics reduced crying, and 6 did not."[cdliv] The concern with results like this is many additional ingredients in probiotics feed the pathogens that cause the problem you are trying to eradicate. Neither the probiotics nor their ingredients were listed in the study.

It is easier to find a probiotic that feeds pathogens than to find a clean product that contains just the probiotic.

The most popular and traditional way to add probiotics into the body is through fermented foods.

In the researched study, overall bowel movements improved, colic dissipated, and regurgitations diminished with the use of probiotics. Crying time for the babies fed the probiotics ranked at 28 minutes, while those who received the placebo cried for 71 minutes each day.

One of the most concerning aspects is vaccinations in these unhealthy babies.

"Vaccinations have been developed for children with a healthy immune system. GAPS children are not fit to be vaccinated with the standard vaccination protocol," says McBride[cdlv]. She lays out a vaccination schedule for these children in her *Gut and Psychology Syndrome* book. The schedule is recommended only after the gut lining is sealed from Leaky Gut and rebuilt with proper probiotic strains.

Non-invasive tests can be done at birth to determine their gut health status. Testing the mother's, father's, and baby's stool and urine can tell you the pathogen overload and future health outlook. If the mother and father have compromised beneficial bacteria in their stool, the baby will have inherited compromised flora. This flora should be rebuilt right from day one, as the studies above show.

Most practitioners agree that a newborn should have consistent rebuilding and training of bacteria with probiotics until they are four years of age. Discontinuing use should not be considered until that time.

The Development of the Infant Microbiome

"The digestive tract is an ideal setting for microbial biofilm formation. It can be considered as a huge bioreactor with a constant temperature, high humidity, regular supply of food and removal of waste. All these are ideal conditions for microbial growth," says Professor Sorensen from the University of Copenhagen, a specialist in microbiology.[cdlvi]

The florae in the intestinal tract serve many functions. They assist in breaking down molecules to use their energy, participate in biosynthesis of vitamins B and K, degrade harmful substances, and keep pathogenic microbes from growing out of control.

Sorensen says, "It is important which microbes we are exposed to and when. A dysbiotic microbiota causes insufficient immune response. The gut microbiota of infants, who would later develop allergy, have been shown to harbor less Enterococcus and Bacteriodes and high amount of Clostridia compared to healthy infants."[cdlvii]

Individuals who develop allergies are shown to have less Bifido and Lactobacillus *bacteria*. They also often present with more Staphylococcus.

"Dysbiosis enhances the risk of development of asthma and other allergic diseases. Diabetes and obesity has been correlated with such dysbiosis," he says.[cdlviii]

Sorensen goes on to say, "Gut colonization may even start before birth through an internal transfer from maternal bacteria to the fetal digestive tract. It is a type of inheritance of maternal microbiota."[cdlix]

The first bacteria to develop in the intestinal tract are Enterobacter, Enterococcus, Lactobacillus, and Streptococcus. The bacteria that colonize in the second phase are Bacteroides, *Bifidibacterium*, Fusobacterium, and Clostridium.

Delivery by cesarean section versus vaginal birth proves less beneficial in developing the balance and healthy population of the infant. Sorensen says, "Children delivered by cesarean section have a two-fold increased risk of developing asthma and other allergic diseases."[cdlx]

In addition to less pathogenic bacteria after birth, infants have shown more beneficial bacteria after birth correlated with mothers who ingested probiotics while pregnant. He says, "The first 1,000 days of life are considered to be the most important period in any individual's life providing the foundation for health. The establishment of a diverse microbiota seems to be a very important factor here."[cdlxi]

The challenge with infant probiotics is the introduction of pathogens through added fillers and binders.

Gates sees success with putting drops of kraut juice into the mouths of infants right after birth.

Supplemental probiotics designed for infants and babies are also beneficial; however, again, be careful of fillers, binders, free-flowing agents, and added ingredients.

Toxic overload in our bodies are higher than ever before, since over 200 toxic chemicals were found in umbilical cord blood of newborn babies. Ken Cook, President of Environmental Working Group (EWG) calls these babies pre-polluted.[cdlxii]

Pre-polluted people.

What is most shocking is that some of these chemicals found have been banned since 1976.

The report entitled "10 Americans" was a comprehensive list of 10 anonymous American newborns and the toxins they contained right from birth. Five different laboratories tested the blood; they found toxins which included mercury, PBTs, PCBs (which the EPA banned in 1976) and, among others, DDT (a pesticide which was also severely limited in 1976).

Scientific American shed light on the report, talking about "the controversial plastics additive Bisphenol A, or BPA, which mimics estrogen and has been shown to cause developmental problems and precancerous growth in animals."[cdlxiii]

Breast Cancer Fund, a breast cancer prevention group, says, "Although the U.S. Environmental Protection Agency banned the use of PCBs in new products in 1976, as many as two-thirds of all PCB containing insulation fluids, plastics, adhesives, paper, inks, paints, dyes and other products manufactured before the ban remain in use today. The remaining one-third was discarded, which means that these toxic compounds eventually made their way into landfills and waste dumps."[cdlxiv]

There are over 300 toxic chemicals in our water that remain unregulated, says Heather White, former General Counsel for EWG, current Executive Director of EWG.[cdlxv]

She also agrees, "Babies are being pre-polluted with toxic chemicals."

Since 2005, she has dedicated her life to shedding light on toxic chemical overload. The "10 Americans" report came out immediately after she delivered her first baby, increasing her awareness of the issue.

White says that these chemicals affect babies, the elderly, and those with autoimmune diseases the hardest. She says, "85% of these chemicals are never tested by the EPA. The companies who make them are not required to test them."[cdlxvi]

Even though the EPA says, "The Safe Drinking Water Act (SDWA) is the main federal law that ensures the quality of Americans' drinking water," a chemical's identity is considered a trade secret.[cdlxvii]

"They won't know anything about the chemical. They don't know where it's manufactured," White says.[cdlxviii] This adds to the problem.

The solution is a high-quality water filter that removes chloride, fluoride, and pesticides. If these items are removed, then the others are captured by default, due to molecular size.

Single-use plastics, like water bottles, are problematic, due to the chemicals that they leach into the water.

They are not recommended for use daily and should only be used in an emergency. White says that their tests show that many bottled waters "are municipal tap water right out of the sink. In many jurisdictions, companies put the tap water in, bottle it and then sell it. It's not very standardized."[cdlxix]

When heated, as happens when the water bottle is sitting in a hot car or in a hot shipping container, these single-use plastic water bottles release BPAs, which add estrogens and other chemicals into the water.

Straws cause the same problems.

Disposable plastic coffee cup lids fall into the same category.

This toxin overload creates the need for probiotics to rebuild the damage.

Parabens and phthalates found in shampoos, lotions, perfumes, and personal care products have also been tested and shown to release estrogens into the body. If the label says *no fragrance* or *no parabens*, but "fragrance" is listed in the ingredients, it contains toxic chemicals that cause damage.

Flame retardants added to mattresses, pillows, and clothing are causing a greater issue as the introduction of these bromides disrupts iodine uptake. Links to hormone disruption, cancer, neurological disorders, and developmental problems are all being blamed on flame retardants. ADHD and mental disturbances are being linked to this low dose exposure.

To make matters worse, *The Chicago Tribune* reported, "When scientists in a government lab touched a small flame to a pair of upholstered chairs — one with a flame retardant in the foam and one without — both were engulfed in flames within four minutes."[cdlxx]

They don't work.

Mercury exposure comes from the air, deposited by manufacturing plants.

Bright red lipsticks contain lead. FDA tests showed 97 percent of over 400 lipsticks tested contained lead.[cdlxxi]

The biggest source of toxins can be ingested through food. The EWG puts together a "clean 15" and "dirty dozen" list every year, listing the most toxic and cleanest foods.

The Toxic Substance Control Act has not been updated since it was established in 1976.

Discrepancies in Food Sources Create Foam in the Stomach and Reproductive Disease

The foods we eat matters. It directly affects our microbiome.

Society is declining in health. This does not just happen without cause. Finding the cause and cleaning up the problem is no small task. Voting with your dollars is a strong and viable force that can change the way products and services are sold. For some who are sick, simply switching their food sources to non-GMO, organic choices is enough to show healing. This fact should not be taken lightly.

Most educated foodies understand the need to avoid GMO foods, pesticides, and herbicides. Many are growing their own vegetables and raising their own livestock on small farms. They are switching their seeds to heirloom seeds, unadulterated seeds, which some say provide optimum flavor and nutrition, since they are in the state in which God made them to nourish.

These savvy foodies are concerned for their health and for the health of their families. Many do so because their kids are horrifically sick. Changing the way their food is made, reverting to food production ways of the early 1900s, has shown incredible healing results in most.

Studies are now surfacing, showing the negative effects of manufactured and altered foods on animals.

"Health concerns long associated with eating beef result not from eating beef, but rather from eating corn-fed beef," says Bill Kiernan, Director at GAI Research & Insight. He goes on to say, "During World War II, farmers were producing more corn than the American population was consuming and so, started feeding the surplus corn to cattle. They soon found that cows eating corn fattened up much quicker than cows eating grass."[cdlxxii]

More importantly, cows are not designed to eat corn. When we change the method of feeding, adverse effects result.

Kiernan says, "A corn diet dangerously raises the acid level in the cow's stomach creating health conditions such as acidosis, necessitating medications and antibiotics which create prime conditions for the existence of *E. Coli*."[cdlxxiii]

The *Merck Veterinarian Manual* says, "Bloat can be a significant cause of mortality in feedlot cattle." They say that bloating comes from grain feed and manifests in two different forms: "Persistent foam mixed with the ruminal contents, called primary or frothy bloat, or in the form of free gas separated from the ingesta."[cdlxxiv]

Nation of Change reported on a recent long-term study exposing the results of GMO feed in cattle and pigs, saying, "Pigs and cows fed on the rather common diet of GMO corn and soy have suffered digestive and reproductive disorders. This is of particular importance since the human digestive tract is very similar to that of pigs."[cdlxxv]

The study used 168 pigs, from birth to slaughter. The pigs were divided into two groups. One was fed GMO corn and soy specifically containing 3 GM proteins, which are herbicides and insecticides.

In detail, they said, "One protein made the plant resistant to a herbicide, and two proteins were insecticides."[cdlxxvi]

The test groups were studied for over 5 months solid while the other was fed an equal, non-GMO diet.

They were taken for processing at the normal slaughter age.[cdlxxvii]

Individuals performing the autopsies were not notified which pigs were fed the GMO diet.

The female pigs fed GMO feed showed numerous health issues including: endometrial hyperplasia, carcinoma, endometriosis, inflammation, thickening of the myometrium, larger presence of polyps, the uteri were fluid-filled, the pigs were 25% larger, inflammation of the stomach and small intestine, stomach ulcers, stomach inflammation, thinning of intestinal walls, and an increase in internal bleeding – specifically, hemorrhaging bowels.[cdlxxviii]

At that same time, *World Truth TV* reported, "The pro-GMO British Environment Secretary, Owen Paterson, has just come out with a major call for the EU to go full-speed ahead with GMO. Paterson told the BBC that GMO crops were 'probably' safer than conventional plants, claiming, without proof, that GMO has significant benefits for farmers, consumers and the environment. He held out the promise that a next generation of GM crops offers the 'most wonderful opportunities to improve human health'."[cdlxxix]

GMO foods are often blamed for having no flavor, as well as for leaving some consumers wanting more food as it doesn't meet the body's requirement for nutrition.

Food is not the only source causing damage to the animals.

Science Blogs reported the study of 153 herds of cattle and 201 herds of deer saying, "High-voltage power lines, which emit strong magnetic fields of their own, disrupt the orientation of cattle and deer. Near these lines, their neat alignment goes astray and they position themselves at random. This disturbance becomes less and less pronounced as the animals stray further away from the power lines."[cdlxxx]

Conversely, Oregon State University tested high voltage power lines with two herds of cattle over 30 months with 205 pairs of cow and calf. They constructed pens directly under the lines. The researchers noted previous studies showed short-term adverse effects were unlikely.[cdlxxxi]

Researchers from Michigan University found different results. Their test showed that suppressed milk production for 3 years recovered after a shield transformer was installed. Behavior also improved. They reported, "Changes of concentrations of several blood and cerebrospinal fluid components, energy and fat metabolism, and reduced milk have been reported for cows exposed to EMF from overhead power lines in Canada. Consequences are related to the time and intensity of exposure to EMF."[cdlxxxii]

Another separate test proved the same negative findings on cattle near EMF. The Institute of Pharmacology, Toxicology and Pharmacology at the Veterinary Faculty of Hannover and the Scientific Institute of Electronics and Radar at the University of the German Federal Armed Forces reported, "Considerable reduction of milk yield and increasing occurrences of health problems, [as well as] behavioral abnormalities that have not yet been examined, have been observed over the last two years in a herd of dairy cows maintained in close proximity to a TV and Radio transmitting antenna."[cdlxxxiii]

They went on to say, "An experiment in which a cow with abnormal behavior was brought to a stable in a different area resulted in normalization of the cow within five days. The symptoms returned, however, when the cow was brought back to the stable in close proximity to the antenna in question. In view of the previously known effects of electromagnetic fields it may be possible that the observed abnormalities are related to the electromagnetic field exposure."[cdlxxxiv]

Martha Herbert, MD, PhD, says that her personal farm reflects the same health issues in her farm animals as in people.[cdlxxxv]

There is something, or many somethings, causing an imbalance in the microbiome across the board. Repair can happen, but it is going to take conscientious effort and diligence. When you support the body correctly, it can repair itself.

Traditionally, societies maintained their health by eating sacred foods that nourished their bodies.

Even today, the average person across the world spends 40 percent of his or her income on food, yet in America, the goal is to spend the least possible on food; for some, this is less than 6 percent of their income. We have the best healthcare system in the world, but we have the sickest people. When you try — try hard — it is nearly impossible to think of someone without any form of illness, allergies, exhaustion, endocrine system disorder, or other disease.

When you support the body, it can repair itself. If it's not food, don't put it in your mouth.

###

About the Author

Nourishing Plot is written by Becky Plotner, ND, traditional naturopath, CGP, D.PSc. who sees clients in Rossville, Georgia. She is a Board Certified Naturopathic Doctor who works as a Certified GAPS Practitioner, seeing clients in her office, via Skype, and on phone. She has been published in *Wise Traditions*, has spoken at two Weston A. Price Conferences and at Certified GAPS Practitioner Trainings, has been on many radio shows and television shows, and writes for Nourishing Plot. Since her son was delivered from the effects of autism (Asperger's syndrome), ADHD, bipolar disorder/manic depression, hypoglycemia and dyslexia, through food, she continued her education, specializing in Leaky Gut and parasitology through Duke University, finishing with distinction. She is a Chapter Leader for The Weston A. Price Foundation.

Discover other titles by Becky Plotner

GAPS, Stage by Stage, with Recipes

Joyous Song, The Proverbs 31 Woman

A Walking Tour of Lincoln Road, South Beach

Ocean Drive Guidebook, Ask a Local

The Fountainebleau, Miami & Los Vegas (Ask a Local)

Connect with Becky Plotner

Blog: https://nourishingplot.com

Website: https://gapsprotocolhelp.com

Facebook: https://www.facebook.com/nourishingplot

Endnotes

---

[i] McBride, Natasha. "GAPS Practitioner Training." Orlando Certified GAPS Practitioner Training Course. Orlando. October 2015. Participatory Lecture.

[ii] McBride, Natasha. *Gut and Psychology Syndrome, Natural Treatment for Autism, Dyspraxia, A.D.D., Dyslexia, A.D.H.D., Depression, Schizophrenia*. Cambridge: Medinform Publishing, 2012. Print.

[iii] Feltman, Rachel. "The Gut's Microbiome Changes Rapidly with Diet." *Scientific American* Dec. 2013: Scientific American. Web. J. 2015.

[iv] Ibid.

[v] Marteau, P, et al. "Metabolism of Bile Salts by Alimentary Bacteria During Transit in the Human Small Intestine." *Microbial Ecology in Health and Disease* Oct. 1994: Taylor & Francis Online. Web. J. 2015.

[vi] Ibid.

[vii] Parvez, S, et al. "Probiotics and their fermented food products are beneficial for health." *Journal of Applied Microbiology* Apr. 2006: Wiley Online Library. Web. J. 2015.

[viii] Ibid.

[ix] Ibid.

[x] Parvez, S. "Probiotics and their fermented food products are beneficial for health." *Journal of Applied Microbiology* Apr. 2006: Wiley Online Library. Web. J. 2015.

[xi] McBride, Natasha. "Gut and Psychology Syndrome (GAPS)." Wise Traditions London. London, England. 2011. Lecture. 41:15.

[xii] Ibid. 41:45.

[xiii] Ibid. 42:15.

[xiv] Ibid. 42:45.

[xv] "Acetaldehyde." https://www.epa.gov/sites/production/files/2016-09/documents/ acetaldehyde.pdf. Dept 2009. PDF File.

[xvi] Ibid.

[xvii] National Center for Biotechnology Information. PubChem Compound Database; CID=177, https://pubchem.ncbi.nlm.nih.gov/compound/177 (accessed Feb. 4, 2017).

[xviii] Ibid.

[xix] Roberts, Carol, et al. "Translocation of Crohn's disease Escherichia coli across M-cells: contrasting effects of soluble plant fibres and emulsifiers." *Gut* Oct. 2010: NCBI. Web. A. 2016.

[xx] Ibid.

[xxi] McBride, Natasha. "The Critical Nature of Gut Health and Its Impact on Children's Brains." The Gluten Summit. Web. 2013. Lecture.

[xxii] Ibid.

[xxiii] Ibid.
[xxiv] Ibid.
[xxv] Ibid.
[xxvi] McBride, Natasha. *Gut and Psychology Syndrome, Natural Treatment for Autism, Dyspraxia, A.D.D., Dyslexia, A.D.H.D., Depression, Schizophrenia*. Cambridge: Medinform Publishing, 2012. Print.
[xxvii] Ibid.
[xxviii] McBride, Natasha. "The Critical Nature of Gut Health and Its Impact on Children's Brains." The Gluten Summit. Web. 2013. Lecture.
[xxix] McBride, Natasha. *Gut and Psychology Syndrome, Natural Treatment for Autism, Dyspraxia, A.D.D., Dyslexia, A.D.H.D., Depression, Schizophrenia.* Cambridge: Medinform Publishing, 2012. Print.
[xxx] McBride, Natasha. "The Critical Nature of Gut Health and Its Impact on Children's Brains." The Gluten Summit. Web. 2013. Lecture.
[xxxi] Ibid.
[xxxii] Yokel, R, et al. "Aluminum bioavailability from basic sodium aluminum phosphate, an approved food additive emulsifying agent, incorporated in cheese." *Food and Chemical Toxicology* June 2008: NCBI Web. Sept. 2016.
[xxxiii] "Natural and Processed Cheese." https://www3.epa.gov/ttnchie1/ap42/ch09/final/c9s06-1.pdf. Dept PDF File.
[xxxiv] Schneider, Andrew. "Test Show Most Store Honey Isn't Honey." *Food and Safety News* Nov. 2011: Food and Safety News Web. Aug. 2015.
[xxxv] Kim, Susanna. "Taco Bell Reveals Its Mystery Beef Ingredients" *ABC News* Apr. 2014: ABCNews.go Web. July 2015.
[xxxvi] Prado, Maria, et al. "Milk kefir: composition, microbial cultures, biological activities, and related products." *Frontiers in Microbiology* Oct. 2015: NCBI Web. Dec. 2015.
[xxxvii] Plotner, Becky. "Surprising Probiotic Count of Kefir Revealed." *Nourishing Plot* Oct. 2015: Nourishing Plot Web. Feb. 2017.
[xxxviii] Ibid.
[xxxix] Ibid.
[xl] Ibid.
[xli] Ibid.
[xlii] Plotner, Becky. "Microbiology Studies Show the Difference Between Store Kefir and Home Brewed Kefir." *Nourishing Plot* Jan. 2016: Nourishing Plot Web. Jan. 2016.
[xliii] Ibid.
[xliv] Ibid.
[xlv] Ibid.
[xlvi] Ibid.
[xlvii] Bolotin, Alexander. "The Complete Genome Sequence of the Lactic Acid Bacterium Lactococcus lactis ssp. lactis IL1403." *Genome Research* May 2001: NCBI Web. Feb. 2015.

[xlviii] Ibid.
[xlix] Muehler, Ashley. "Lactococcus lactis." *Microbe of The Week* 2009: Web.mst.edu Web. June 2015.
[l] Yang, Chun, et al. "Bacteremia Due to Vancomycin-Resistant Leuconostoc lactis in a Patient with Pneumonia and Abdominal Infection." *The American Journal of Medical Sciences* March 2015: NCBI Web. May 2015.
[li] McBride, Natasha. "Gut and Psychology Syndrome." Annual Wise Traditions Conference. Anaheim, California. 2015. Lecture.
[lii] "Pandas Frequently Asked Questions." National Institute of Mental Health: NIMH Web. Aug. 2015.
[liii] Ibid.
[liv] Tahmourespour, Arezoo and Rooha Kasra Kermanshahi, "The effect of a probiotic strain (Lactobacillus acidophilus) on the plaque formation of oral Streptococci." *Bosnian Journal of Basic Medical Sciences* Feb. 2011: NCBI Web. July 2015.
[lv] Ibid.
[lvi] Wolfson, David, et al. "PANDAS, Autism Spectrum Disorders and Involvement of Streptococcus Organisms." Klaire Labs, Technical Studies: Klaire Web. Aug. 2015.
[lvii] Ibid.
[lviii] Trojanova, Iva and Vojtech Rada. "Enzymatic Activity in Fermented Milk Products Containing Bifidobacteria." *Czech Journal of Food Science* Vol 23, No. 6: 224-229: Architecture Journals Web. Oct. 2015.
[lix] LeBlanc, JG, et al. "Bacteria as vitamin suppliers to their host: a gut microbiota perspective." *Current Opinion in Biotechnology* April 2013: NCBI Web. Jan. 2015.
[lx] Thantsha, M.S., C.I. Mamvura and J. Booyens. "Probiotics – What They Are, Their Benefits and Challenges." *Intech*: Intech Web. Dec. 2016.
[lxi] Barreau, Claude and Georges Wagener. "Characterization of Leuconostoc lactis Strains from Human Sources." *Journal of Clinical Microbiology* Aug. 1990: NCBI Web. Sept. 2015.
[lxii] Jenney, A. "Enterococcus durans." *Journal of Antimicrobial Chemotherapy* Sept. 2000: Oxford Academic Web. Aug. 2015.
[lxiii] "DNA repair protein RadA." *Uniprot*: Uniprot.org Web. Sept. 2015.
[lxiv] LINARES, Daniel M. et al. "The tyrosyl-tRNA synthetase like gene located in the tyramine biosynthesis cluster of Enterococcus duransis transcriptionally regulated by tyrosine concentration and extracellular pH." *BMC Microbiology* Feb. 2012: bmcmicrobioal.biomedcentral Web. July 2015.
[lxv] Raspor, P and D. Goranovic. "Biotechnological applications of acetic acid bacteria." *Critical Reviews in Biotechnology* Oct. 2008: Taylor & Francis Online Web. Jan. 2015.
[lxvi] Plotner, Becky. "Microbiology Studies Show the Difference Between Store Kefir and Home Brewed Kefir." *Nourishing Plot* Jan. 2016: Nourishing Plot Web. Jan. 2016.

[lxvii] Ibid.
[lxviii] Ibid.
[lxix] Ibid.
[lxx] Ibid.
[lxxi] Ibid.
[lxxii] Ibid.
[lxxiii] McBride, Natasha. *Gut and Psychology Syndrome, Natural Treatment for Autism, Dyspraxia, A.D.D., Dyslexia, A.D.H.D., Depression, Schizophrenia.* Cambridge: Medinform Publishing, 2012. Print.
[lxxiv] Chen, H. -L. et al. "Kefir improves bone mass and microarchitecture in an ovariectomized rat model of postmenopausal osteoporosis." *Osteoporosis International* Oct. 2014: Springer Link Web. Dec. 2014.
[lxxv] Ibid. February 2015, Volume 26, Issue 2, pp 589-599.
[lxxvi] Katayama, Kou et al. "Supplemental treatment of rheumatoid arthritis with natural milk antibodies against enteromicrobes and their toxins: results of an open-labeled pilot study." *Nutrition Journal* Jan. 2011: Nutritionjournal.biomendcentral Web. June 2015.
[lxxvii] Ibid.
[lxxviii] Ibid.
[lxxix] Rossel, Jose. "Yoghourt and kefir in their relation to health and therapeutics." *Canadian Medical Association Journal* March 1932: NCBI Web. Feb. 2015.
[lxxx] Guzel-Swydim, Z, et al. "Effect of different growth conditions on biomass increase in kefir grains." The Journal of Dairy Science Mar. 2011: journalofdairyscience.org Web. April 2015.
[lxxxi] Amiri Roudbar, Mahamoud, et al. "Estimates of variance components due to parent-of-origin effects for body weight in Iran-Black sheep." *Small Ruminant Research* Dec. 2015: Science Direct Web. Dec. 2015.
[lxxxii] Ibid.
[lxxxiii] Noori, Negin, et al., "Kefir protective effects against nicotine cessation-induced anxiety and cognition impairments in rats." *Advanced Biomedical Research* Dec. 2014: NCBI Web. Aug. 2015.
[lxxxiv] Ibid.
[lxxxv] Ibid.
[lxxxvi] Ibid.
[lxxxvii] Hertzler, SR and SM Clancy. "Kefir improves lactose digestion and tolerance in adults with lactose maldigestion." *Journal of the Academy of Nutrition and Dietetics* Mar. 2003: andjrnl Web. Oct. 2015.
[lxxxviii] "Kefir May Bolster Lactose in Intolerant People." *Science Daily* Mar. 2003: Science Daily Web. June 2015.
[lxxxix] Ibid.
[xc] Kudret Adiloglu, Ali, et al, "The Effect of Kefir Consumption on Human Immune System: A Cytokine Study." *Bulletin of Microbiology* July 2013: mikrobiyolbul Web. Sept. 2015.

[xci] Ibid.

[xcii] Farnworth, Edward. (2006). "Kefir – A Complex Probiotic." *Food Science and Technology Bulletin*, vol. 2, 1-17. https://books.google.com/books?id=nn2-lqEXdqcC&pg=PA14&lpg=PA14&dq=Kwak,+H.S.,+Park,+S.K.,+Kim,+D.+S. +(1996)+Biostabilization+of+kefir+with+a+non-lactose+fermenting+yeast.+Journal+of+Dairy+Science+79:937942.&source=bl&ots=ri9a2Ckpt-&sig=lmUGq2axjFaZX302ili32L-Jk7E&hl=en&sa=X&ved=0ahUKEwjT6sHVj6rNAhWK1CYKHX9EC1oQ6AEIHjAB#v=onepage&q=Kwak%2C%20H.S.%2C%20Park%2C%20S.K.%2C%20Kim%2C%20D.%20S.%20(1996)%20Biostabilization%20of%20kefir%20with%20a%20nonlactose%20fermenting%20yeast.%20Journal%20of%20Dairy%20Science%2079%3A937-942.&f=false

[xciii] Ibid. p. 12.

[xciv] O'Brien, K.V., et al. "The effects of frozen storage on the survival of probiotic microorganisms found in traditionally and commercially manufactured kefir." *Journal of Dairy Science* Sept. 2016: Journal of Dairy Science Web. Dec. 2016.

[xcv] Young, Ed. "Breast-feeding the microbiome." *The New Yorker* July 2016: thenewyorker Web. Sept. 2016.

[xcvi] Ibid.

[xcvii] Ibid.

[xcviii] O'Brien, Keely Virginia. (May 2012) The effect of frozen storage on the survival of probiotic microorganisms found in traditional and commercial kefir (master's thesis). Retrieved from Louisiana State University docs database (http://etd.lsu.edu/docs/available/etd-04252012-155457/unrestricted/obrien-thesis.pdf.)

[xcix] O'Brien, K.V., et al. "The effects of frozen storage on the survival of probiotic microorganisms found in traditionally and commercially manufactured kefir." *Journal of Dairy Science* Sept. 2016: Journal of Dairy Science Web. Dec. 2016.

[c] Ibid.

[ci] Ibid.

[cii] Ibid.

[ciii] Ibid.

[civ] Ibid.

[cv] Farnworth, Edward. (2006). "Kefir – A Complex Probiotic." *Food Science and Technology Bulletin*, vol. 2, 11. https://books.google.com/books?id=nn2-lqEXdqcC&pg=PA14&lpg=PA14&dq=Kwak,+H.S.,+Park,+S.K.,+Kim,+D.+S.+(1996)+Biostabilization+of+kefir+with+a+non-lactose+fermenting+yeast.+Journal+of+Dairy+Science+79:937942.&source=bl&ots=ri9a2Ckpt-&sig=lmUGq2axjFaZX302ili32L-Jk7E&hl=en&sa=X&ved=0ahUKEwjT6sHVj6rNAhWK1CYKHX9EC1oQ6AEIHjAB#v=onepage&q=Kwak%2C%20H.S.%2C%20Park%2C%20S.K.%2C%20Kim%2C%20D.%20S.%20(1996)%20Biostabilization%20of%20kefir%20with%20a%20nonlactose%20fermenting%20yeast.%2

0Journal%20of%20Dairy%20Science%2079%3A937-942.&f=false
[cvi] Rosell, Jose. "Yoghourt and kefir in their relation to health and therapeutics." Canadian Medical Association Mar. 2013: NCBI Web. Sept. 2016.
[cvii] Ibid.
[cviii] Ibid.
[cix] Ibid.
[cx] Ibid.
[cxi] Ibid.
[cxii] Ibid.
[cxiii] Ibid.
[cxiv] Ibid.
[cxv] Ibid.
[cxvi] Ibid.
[cxvii] Ibid.
[cxviii] Plotner, Becky. "Microbiology Studies Show the Difference Between Store Kefir and Home Brewed Kefir." *Nourishing Plot* Jan. 2016: Nourishing Plot Web. Jan. 2016.
[cxix] Ibid.
[cxx] Ibid.
[cxxi] Rosell, Jose. "Yoghourt and kefir in their relation to health and therapeutics." *Canadian Medical Association* Mar. 2013: NCBI Web. Sept. 2016. Page 344.
[cxxii] Elli, Marina, et al. "Survival of Yogurt Bacteria in the Human Gut." *Applied and Environmental Microbiology* July 2006: NCBI Web. Sept. 2016.
[cxxiii] "Milk Facts.": *Milk Facts Info* Web. Dec. 2016. http://milkfacts.info/Milk%20Processing/Yogurt%20Production.html
[cxxiv] Hixson, Mary. "Probiotics in the prevention of antibiotic-associated diarrhea and Clostridium difficile infection." *Therapeutic Advances in Gastroenterology* May 2011: NCBI Web. July 2016.
[cxxv] Martini, M.C., et al. "Strains and species of lactic acid bacteria in fermented milks (yogurts): effect on in vivo lactose digestion." *The American Journal of Clinical Nutrition* Dec. 1991: ajcn.nutrition Web. Oct 2015.
[cxxvi] Jusuf, Moshood A. and Tengku Haziyamin Abdul Tengku Abdul Hamid. "Lactic Acid Bacteria: Bacteriocin Producer: A Mini Review." *IOSR Journal of Pharmacy* May 2013: iosrphr Web. Sept. 2015.
[cxxvii] Tahmourespour, Arezoo and Rooha Kasra Kermanshahi. "The effect of a probiotic strain (Lactobacillus acidophilus) on the plaque formation of oral Streptococci." Bosnian Journal of Basic Medical Sciences Feb. 2011: NCBI Web. July 2015.
[cxxviii] "Lactobacillus." *MedlinePlus*: MedlinePlus Web. Nov. 2016.
[cxxix] Barnard, Neal. *Power Foods for The Brain* New York: Grand Central Lifestyle.
[cxxx] "The effect of vitamin E and beta carotene on the incidence of lung cancer and other cancers in male smokers. The Alpha-Tocopherol, Beta Carotene Cancer Prevention Study Group." New England Journal of Medicine April 1994:

NCBI Web. Sept. 2015.

[cxxxi] DeNoon, Daniel J. "Death Stalks Smokers in Beta-Carotene Study Years After Smokers Stop Beta-Carotene Supplements, Lung Cancer Deaths Up." WebMD Nov. 2004: WebMD Web. July 2016.

[cxxxii] Barnard, Neal. *Power Foods for The Brain* New York: Grand Central Lifestyle.

[cxxxiii] Ibid.

[cxxxiv] DeNoon, Daniel J. "Death Stalks Smokers in Beta-Carotene Study Years After Smokers Stop Beta-Carotene Supplements, Lung Cancer Deaths Up." WebMD Nov. 2004: WebMD Web. July 2016.

[cxxxv] "The Effect of Vitamin E and Beta Carotene on The Incidence of Lung Cancer in Male Smokers." *The New England Journal of Medicine* April 1994: NEJM Web. Feb. 2015.

[cxxxvi] Barnard, Neal. *Power Foods for The Brain* New York: Grand Central Lifestyle.

[cxxxvii] Ibid.

[cxxxviii] Ibid.

[cxxxix] Barnard, Neal. Physicians Committee of Responsible Medicine: pcrm.org Web. Nov. 2014.

[cxl] "Health Concerns about Dairy Products." Physicians Committee for Responsible Medicine: pcrm.org Web Aug. 2015.

[cxli] Tang, Mimi L.K., et al. "Administration of a probiotic with peanut oral immunotherapy: A randomized trial." *The Journal of Allergy and Clinical Immunology* March 2015: joacionline Web. Oct. 2015.

[cxlii] Bushak, Lecia. "Oral Immunotherapy Combination of Peanut Protein, Probiotics May Cure Peanut Allergies." *Medical Daily* Jan. 2015: medicaldaily Web. Feb. 2015.

[cxliii] Canani, Robert Berni, et al., "The Potential Therapeutic Efficacy of Lactobacillus GG in Children with Food Allergies." *Pharmaceuticals* June 2012: NCBI Web. Feb. 2015.

[cxliv] Ibid.

[cxlv] Reid, Gregor. "Probiotics for Women's Health: The Story of Lactobacillus Rhamnosus GR-1 and Lactobacillus Reuteri RC-14." *Superior Nutrition and Formulation Jarrow Formulas*: Jarrow.com Web. Aug. 2016.

[cxlvi] Ibid.

[cxlvii] Sanchez, M. "Effect of Lactobacillus rhamnosus CGMCC1.3724 supplementation on weight loss and maintenance in obese men and women." *The British Journal of Nutrition* April 2014: NCBI Web. Feb. 2015.

[cxlviii] Molin, Goran. "Probiotics in foods not containing mik or milk constituents, with special reference to Lactobacillus plantarum 299v." *The American Journal of Clinical Nutrition Feb.* 2001: ajcn.nutrition Web. Jan. 2015.

[cxlix] "Man suffering from constipation for 10 years has 11-pound stool removed." Fox Health News Aug. 2015: foxnews.com Web. Dec. 2016.

[cl] Mercola, Joseph. 2008: (September 8). Dr. Mercola Interviews Dr. Stephanie Seneff (part 1). Retrieved from

https://www.youtube.com/watch?v=5QUChSlUEH0
[cli] Ibid.
[clii] Ibid.
[cliii] Mazlyn, M.M., et al. "Effects of a probiotic fermented milk on functional constipation: a randomized, double-blind, placebo-controlled study." *Journal of Gastroenterology and Hepatology* July 2013: NCBI Web. Jan. 2015.
[cliv] Sadeghzadeh, M., et al. "The Effect of Probiotics on Childhood Constipation: A Randomized Controlled Double Blind Clinical Trial." *International Journal of Pediatrics* Apr. 2014: hindawi Web. Mar. 2015.
[clv] Ibid.
[clvi] Ibid.
[clvii] Beausoleil, M. "Effect of a fermented milk combining Lactobacillus acidophilus CI1285 and Lactobacillus casei in the prevention of antibiotic-associated diarrhea: a randomized, double-blind, placebo-controlled trial." *Canadian Journal of Gastorenterology* Nov. 2007: NCBI Web. Dec. 2014.
[clviii] Corinna Koebnick, Irmtrud Wagner, Peter Leitzmann, Udo Stern, and HJ Franz Zunft, "Probiotic Beverage Containing Lactobacillus casei Shirota Improves Gastrointestinal Symptoms in Patients with Chronic Constipation," Canadian Journal of Gastroenterology, vol. 17, no. 11, pp. 655-659, 2003. https://doi.org/10.1155/2003/654907.
[clix] Khodadad, Ahmad, et al., "Role of Synbiotics in the Treatment of Childhood Constipation: A Double-Blind Randomized Placebo Controlled Trial." *Iranian Journal of Pediatrics* Dec. 2010: NCBI Web. Feb. 2015.
[clx] Takeda, Guarantor M. "The effect of Lactobacillus helveticus fermented milk on sleep and health perception in elderly subjects." *European Journal of Clinical Nutrition* Sept. 2007: nature.com Web. Aug. 2016.
[clxi] Songisepp, Epp., et al. "Evaluation of the functional efficacy of an antioxidative probiotic in healthy volunteers." *Nutrition Journal Aug.* 2005: NCBI Web. Feb. 2015.
[clxii] Jayasimhana, Sanmugapriya, et al., "Efficacy of microbial cell preparation in improving chronic constipation: A randomized, double-blind, placebo-controlled trial." *Clinical Nutrition* Dec. 2013: ScienceDirect Web. Feb. 2015.
[clxiii] Guerra, Paula VP, et al. "Pediatric functional constipation treatment with Bifidobacterium-containing yogurt: A crossover, double-blind, controlled trial." *World Journal of Gastroenterology* Sept. 2011: NCBI Web. Feb. 2015.
[clxiv] Miller, Larry E., and Arthur C. Ouwehand. "Probiotic supplementation decreases intestinal transit time: Meta-analysis of randomized controlled trials." *World Journal of Gastroenterology* Aug. 2013: NCBI Web. Feb. 2015.
[clxv] Saneian, Hossein, et. al. "Comparison of Lactobacillus Sporogenes plus mineral oil and mineral oil alone in the treatment of childhood functional constipation." *The Journal of Research in Medical Sciences* Jan. 2013: jrms.mui.ac.ir Web. Feb. 2015.
[clxvi] Mazlyn, Mena Mustapha, et al. "Effects of a Probiotic Fermented Milk on

Functional Constipation, A Randomized, Double-blind, Placebo-Controlled Study." *Journal of Gastroenterology and Hepatology July* 2013: Medscape Web. Feb. 2015.
[clxvii] Ibid.
[clxviii] Mercola, Joseph. 2013: (August 28). Dr. Mercola Interviews Sandor Katz About Fermentation. Retrieved from https://www.youtube.com/watch?v=LkXT-XgyzkI
[clxix] Ibid.
[clxx] Ibid.
[clxxi] McBride, Natasha. "The Critical Nature of Gut Health and Its Impact on Children's Brains." The Gluten Summit. Web. 2013. Lecture.
[clxxii] Ibid.
[clxxiii] Ibid.
[clxxiv] Rettner, Rachael. "'Autistic' Mice Help Researchers Study Disorder." *Live Science* Sept. 2011: Live Science Web. Feb. 2015.
[clxxv] "Mice With 'Mohawks' Help Researchers Get to The Biological Bottom of Autism." *HNGN* May 2014: HNGN Web. Feb. 2015.
[clxxvi] Karayannis, T, et al. "Mice with 'mohawks' help scientists link autism to two biological pathways in brain." *Science Daily* May 2014: ScienceDaily Web. Feb. 2015.
[clxxvii] Ibid.
[clxxviii] "Mice With 'Mohawks' Help Researchers Get to The Biological Bottom of Autism," *HNGN* May 2014: HNGN Web. Feb. 2015.
[clxxix] "GABA (Gamma-Aminobutyric Acid)." WebMD: WebMD Web. Feb. 2015.
[clxxx] Sugiyama T., and Y. Sadzuka. "GABA: Gamma-Amino Butyric Acid." DNC News: Denver Naturopathic Clinic Web. Feb. 2015.
[clxxxi] Ibid.
[clxxxii] Inoue, K., et al. "GABA Lo-Do Internal Medicine." *Texmedsals.biz* July 2016: Texmedsals.biz Web. Feb. 2015.
[clxxxiii] "GABA." therapy.epnet: therapy.epnet Web. Feb. 2015.
[clxxxiv] McBride, Natasha. *Gut and Psychology Syndrome, Natural Treatment for Autism, Dyspraxia, A.D.D., Dyslexia, A.D.H.D., Depression, Schizophrenia.* Cambridge: Medinform Publishing, 2012. Print.
[clxxxv] Ibid.
[clxxxvi] "GABA." therapy.epnet: therapy.epnet Web. Feb. 2015.
[clxxxvii] McBride, Natasha. "Gut and Psychology Syndrome." Annual Wise Traditions Conference. Anaheim, California. 2015. Lecture.
[clxxxviii] Deans, Emily. "Groovy Probiotics." *Psychology Today* June 2012: psychologytoday Web. Feb. 2015.
[clxxxix] Enwa, Felix O., "A mini review on the microbiochemical properties of sauerkraut." *African Journal of Science and Research* Jan. 2014: ajsr.rstpublishers Web. Feb. 2015.
[cxc] McBride, Natasha. "Gut and Psychology Syndrome." Annual Wise Traditions

Conference. Anaheim, California. 2015. Lecture.
[cxci] Katz, Sandor Ellix. *Wild Fermentation: The Flavor, Nutrition, and Craft of Live-Culture Foods Reclaiming Domesticity form a Consumer Culture.* Vermont: Chelsey Green Publishing, 2003. Print.
[cxcii] Mercola, Joseph. 2013: (August 28). Dr. Mercola Interviews Sandor Katz About Fermentation. Retrieved from https://www.youtube.com/watch?v=LkXT-XgyzkI
[cxciii] Siebecker, Allison. "Small Intestinal Bacteria Overgrowth." The Healthy Gut Summit. Web. 2015. Lecture.
[cxciv] Ibid.
[cxcv] Mercola, Joseph. 2011: (December 20). Dr. Mercola Interviews Dr. Natasha Campbell-McBride. Retrieved from https://www.youtube.com/watch?v=bYJkS3ZBqos (30:50).
[cxcvi] Mercola, Joseph. 2014: (June 16). Take Control of Your Health! With Joseph Mercola, DO. Retrieved from https://www.youtube.com/watch?v=v5KB_2j3nuI (53:20).
[cxcvii] Godfrey, Susan. "Study of Microbial Succession in Fermenting Cabbage." *Council on Undergraduate Research*: cur.org Web. Jan. 2017.
[cxcviii] Ibid.
[cxcix] Ibid.
[cc] Lu, Z., et al. "Bacteriophage Ecology in Commercial Sauerkraut Fermentations." *Applied and Environmental Microbiology* June 2003: aem.asm Web. Feb. 2015.
[cci] Fleming, H.P., et al. "A Fermenter for Study of Sauerkraut Fermentation." Department of Food, Bioprocessing & Nutrition Sciences Jan. 1987: fbns.ncsu.edu Web. Feb. 2015.
[ccii] Smith, Leonard. "The Gut Microbiome: Pregnancy and Childhood." The Healthy Gut Summit. Web. 2015. Lecture.
[cciii] Ibid.
[cciv] Ibid.
[ccv] Ibid.
[ccvi] Ibid.
[ccvii] Ibid.
[ccviii] Lahti, Leo, et al. "Associations between the human intestinal microbiota, Lactobacillus rhamnosus GG and serum lipids indicated by integrated analysis of high-throughput profiling data." *PeerJ* Aug. 2015: peerj.com Web. Oct. 2015.
[ccix] Poutahidis, Theofilos, et al. "Probiotic Microbes Sustain Youthful Serum Testosterone Levels and Testicular Size in Aging Mice." *PLoS One* Jan. 2014: NCBI Web. Feb. 2016.
[ccx] Bhandar, Praveen, et al. "Potential of Probiotic Lactobacillus plantarum 2621 for the Management of Infertility." *British Microbiology Research Journal* Dec. 2014: sciencedomain.org Web. Feb. 2015.
[ccxi] Barton-Schuster, Dalene. "Fertility Health Tip: Probiotics and Prebiotics."

Natural Fertility Info.: natural-fertility-info Web. Feb. 2015.

[ccxii] Uchida, M. and O. Kobayashi. "Effects of Lactobacillus gaseri OLL2809 on the induced endometriosis in rats." *Bioscience, Biotechnology, and Biochemistry Sept.* 2013: NCBI Web. Feb. 2015.

[ccxiii] Itoh, H, et al. "Lsctobacillus gasseri OLL2809 is effective especially on the menstrual pain and dysmenorrhea in endometriosis patients: randomized, double-blind, placebo-controlled study." *Cytotechnology* Mar. 2011: NCBI Web. Feb. 2015.

[ccxiv] Weng, SL., et al. "Bacterial communities in semes from men of infertile couples: metagenomic sequencing reveals relationships of seminal microbiota to semen quality." *PLoS One* Oct. 2014: NCBI Web. Feb. 2015.

[ccxv] Smith, Leonard. "The Gut Microbiome: Pregnancy and Childhood." The Healthy Gut Summit. Web. 2015. Lecture.

[ccxvi] Gates, Donna. "Cracking the Code on the Gut-Gene Connection." The Healthy Gut Summit. Web. 2015. Lecture.

[ccxvii] McBride, Natasha. "Gut and Psychology Syndrome." Annual Wise Traditions Conference. Anaheim, California. 2015. Lecture.

[ccxviii] Cho, K.M, et al. "Biodegredation of chlorpyrifos by lactic acid bactria during kimchi fermentation." *Journal of Agriculture and Food Chemistry* Mar. 2011: NCBI Web. Feb. 2015.

[ccxix] Cheigh, Hong-Sik, et al. "Biochemical, microbiological, and nutritional aspects of kimchi (Korean fermented vegetable products)." *Critical Reviews in Food Science and Nutrition* Sept. 2009: tandfonline Web. Feb. 2015.

[ccxx] Ibid.

[ccxxi] Rhee, Sook Jong, et al. "Importance of lactic acid bacteria in Asian fermented foods." *Microbial Cell Factories* Aug. 2011: microbialcellfactories.biomed Web. Feb. 2015.

[ccxxii] Choi, In Hwa, et al. "Kimchi, a Fermented Vegetable, Improves Serum Lipid Profiles in Healthy Young Adults: Randomized Clinical Trial." *Journal of Medicinal Food* Mar. 2013: NCBI Web. Feb. 2015.

[ccxxiii] Ibid.

[ccxxiv] Kim, Hyun Ju, et al. "Effect of kimchi intake on lipid profiles and blood pressure." *Kidney Research and Clinical Practice* June 2012: sciencedirect Web. Feb. 2015.

[ccxxv] Lee, Seung-Min, et al. "Effects of kimchi supplementation on blood pressure and cardiac hypertrophy with varying sodium content in spontaneously hypertensive rats." *Nutrition Research and Practice* Aug. 2012: NCBI Web. Feb. 2015.

[ccxxvi] Kim, E.K., et al. "Fermented kimchi reduces body weight and improves metabolic parameters in overweight and obese patients." *Nutrition Research* Jun. 2011: NCBI Web. Feb. 2015.

[ccxxvii] Ibid.

[ccxxviii] "The health benefits of kimchi" *Fox News* June 2016: FoxNews Web. Feb. 2015.

[ccxxix] Chu, Michael and Terry F. Seltzer. "Myxedema Coma Induced by Ingestion

of Raw Bok Choy." *New England Journal of Medicine* May 2010: nejm.com Web. Jan. 2015.
[ccxxx] Ibid.
[ccxxxi] Ibid.
[ccxxxii] Ibid.
[ccxxxiii] Ibid.
[ccxxxiv] Adams, Duncan. "Deliverance from exophthalmic goiter deaths." *New Zealand Journal of Medicine* May 2011: nzma.org.nz Web. Jan. 2015.
[ccxxxv] Ibid.
[ccxxxvi] Hummel, Barbara. "Top 10 Doctor insights on: What Does A Palpable Thyroid Mean, What Should You Eat When You Have Hyperthyroidism." *HealthTap*: Healthtap Web. Oct. 2016.
[ccxxxvii] Weil, Andrew. "Is broccoli bad for the thyroid?" Weil June 2005: drweil.com Web. Jan. 2015.
[ccxxxviii] Nguyen, Nguyen Khoi, et al. "Lactic acid bacteria: promising supplements for enhancing the biological activities of kombucha." Feb. 2015: *SpringerPlus* Web. Aug. 2015.
[ccxxxix] Ibid.
[ccxl] Ibid.
[ccxli] Ibid.
[ccxlii] Ibid.
[ccxliii] Misra, Suniti, et al. "Utilization of Glycosaminoglycans/Proteoglycans as Carriers for Targeted Therapy Delivery." *International Journal of Cell* Biology Sept. 2015: NCBI Web. Nov. 2015.
[ccxliv] Barati, Fardin, et al. "Histopathological and clinical evaluation of Kombucha tea and Nitrofurazone on cutaneous full thickness wounds healing in rats: an experimental study." *Diagnostic Pathology* July 2013: diagnosticpathology.biomedcentral Web. Nov. 2015.
[ccxlv] Ibid.
[ccxlvi] Ibid.
[ccxlvii] Ibid.
[ccxlviii] Ibid.
[ccxlix] Velicanski, Aleksandra S., et al., "Antimicrobial and antioxidant activity of lemon balm Kombucha." *Acta Periodica Technologica* 2007: scindeks.ceon.rs Web. Nov. 2015.
[ccl] Nguyen, Nguyen Khoi, et al. "Lactic acid bacteria: promising supplements for enhancing the biological activities of kombucha." Feb. 2015: *SpringerPlus* Web. Aug. 2015.
[ccli] Ibid.
[cclii] Rashid, Kahkashan, et al., "Protective role of D-saccharic acid-1, 4-.actone in alloxan induced oxidative stress in the spleen tissue of diabetic rats in mediated by suppressing mitochondria dependent apoptotic pathway." *Free Radical Research* Jan. 2012: tandfonline Web. Nov. 2015.

[ccliii] "Niacin and niacinamide (Vitamin B3)." *Medline Plus*: medlineplus.gov Web. Nov. 2015.
[ccliv] Bauer, Brent. "What is Kombucha tea? Does it have any health benefits?" Mayo Clinic June 2014: mayoclinic.org Web. Nov. 2015.
[cclv] Ibid.
[cclvi] "Unexplained Severe Illness Possibly Associated with Consumption of Kombucha Tea -- Iowa, 1995." *MMWR Weekly* Dec. 1995: cdc.gov Web. Oct. 2015.
[cclvii] Ibid.
[cclviii] Ibid.
[cclix] Ibid.
[cclx] Ibid.
[cclxi] Ibid.
[cclxii] Ibid.
[cclxiii] Ibid.
[cclxiv] Ibid.
[cclxv] Ibid.
[cclxvi] Ibid.
[cclxvii] Ibid.
[cclxviii] Ibid.
[cclxix] Mosiehj-Jenabian, Saloomeh, et al. "Beneficial Effects of Probiotics and Food Borne Yeasts on Human Health." *Nutrients* Apr. 2010: NCBI Web. Nov. 2015.
[cclxx] Ibid.
[cclxxi] Kelesidis, Theodoros and Charalabos Pothoulakjs. "Efficacy and safety of the probiotic Saccharomyces boulardii for the prevention and therapy of gastrointestinal disorders." *Therapeutic Advances in Gastroenterology* Mar. 2012: NCBI Web. Jan. 2015.
[cclxxii] Mann U, "Verbluffend - ein Pilz Kuriert den Darm", Bild und Funk, 35, 1988.
[cclxxiii] Chakravortya, Somnath, et al. "Kombucha tea fermentation: Microbial and biochemical dynamics." *International Journal of Food Microbiology* Mar. 2016: Science Direct Web. Nov. 2015.
[cclxxiv] Ibid.
[cclxxv] Ibid.
[cclxxvi] Ibid.
[cclxxvii] Correa dos Santos, Renato Augusto, et al. "Draft Genome Sequence of Komagataeibacter intermedium Strain AF2, a Producer of Cellulose, Isolated from Kombucha Tea." *Genome Announcements* Dec. 2015: genome.asm.org Web. Dec. 2015.
[cclxxviii] Ibid.
[cclxxix] Chakravorty, S, et al. "Identification of new conserved and variable regions in the 16S rRNA gene of acetic acid bacteria and acetobacteraceae family." *Molekuliarnaia Biologiia* Oct. 2015: NCBI Web. Nov. 2015.

[cclxxx] Watawana, Mindani, et al. "Application of the Kombucha 'tea fungus' for the enhancement of antioxidant and starch hydrolase inhibitory properties of ten herbal teas." *Food Chemistry* Mar. 2016: Science Direct Web. June 2016.
[cclxxxi] Ibid.
[cclxxxii] Ibid.
[cclxxxiii] Lobo, R.O. and C.K. Shenoy. "Myocardial potency of Bio-tea against Isoproterenol induced myocardial damage in rats." *Journal of Food Science and Technology* Jul. 2015: NCBI Web. Aug. 2015.
[cclxxxiv] Ibid.
[cclxxxv] Bellassoued, Khaled, et al. "Protective effect of Kombucha on rats fed a hypercholesterolemic diet is mediated by its antioxidant activity." *Pharmaceutical Biology* May 2015: tandfonline Web. June 2015.
[cclxxxvi] Ibid.
[cclxxxvii] Ibid.
[cclxxxviii] Chakravortya, Somnath, et al. "Kombucha tea fermentation: Microbial and biochemical dynamics." *International Journal of Food Microbiology Mar.* 2016: Science Direct Web. April 2016.
[cclxxxix] Rashid, Kahkashan, et al., "Protective role of D-saccharic acid-1, 4-.actone in alloxan induced oxidative stress in the spleen tissue of diabetic rats in mediated by suppressing mitochondria dependent apoptotic pathway." *Free Radical Research* Jan. 2012: tandfonline Web. Nov. 2015.
[ccxc] Ibid.
[ccxci] Marzban, Fatemeh, et al. "Kombucha tea ameliorates experimental encephalomyelitis in mouse of multiple sclerosis." *Food and Agricultural Immunology* Sept. 2014: tandfonline Web. June 2015.
[ccxcii] Ibid.
[ccxciii] Murugesan, G.S., et al. "Hepatoprotective and Curative Properties of Kombucha Tea Against Carbon Tetrachloride- Induced Toxicity." *Journal of Microbiology and Biotechnology* Dec. 2008: jmb.or.kr Web. Aug. 2015.
[ccxciv] Greenwalt, C.J., et al. "Kombucha, the Fermented Tea: Microbiology, Composition, and Claimed Health Effects." *Journal of Food Protection* July 2000: ingenntacommect Web. Aug. 2015.
[ccxcv] Aloulou, A, et al. "Hypoglycemic and antilipidemic properties of Kombucha tea in alloxan-induced diabetic rats." *BMC Complementary and Alternative Medicine* May 2012: NCBI Web. Aug. 2015.
[ccxcvi] Ibid.
[ccxcvii] Bollinger, Ty. "Interview with Dr. Patrick Vikers." The Truth About Cancer. Web. 2015. Lecture.
[ccxcviii] Ibid.
[ccxcix] Ibid.
[ccc] Ibid.
[ccci] Fallon, Sally and Mary Enig. *Nourishing Traditions* Washington: New Trends Publishing, 1999. Print.

[cccii] Sacks, Katherine. (2015, July). Why Does Garlic Turn Blue? *Epicurious.* https://www.epicurious.com/expert-advice/why-does-garlic-turn-blue-article.
[ccciii] Jung, Young-Mi, et al. "Fermented garlic protects diabetic, obese mice when fed a high-fat diet by antioxidant effects." *Nutrition Research* May 2011: nrjournal Web. June 2015.
[ccciv] Sato, Emiko, et al. "Increased Anti-oxidative Potency of Garlic by Spontaneous Short-term Fermentation." *Plant Foods for Human Nutrition* Dec. 2006: link.springer Web. Aug. 2015.
[cccv] Ibid.
[cccvi] Ibid.
[cccvii] Yan, L and H. Kim. "Effects of dietary supplementation of fermented garlic powder on growth performance, apparent total tract digestibility, blood characteristics and faecal microbial concentration in weaning pigs." *Animal Physiology and Animal Nutrition* Mar. 2012: onlinelibrary.wiley Web. Feb. 2015.
[cccviii] Ibid.
[cccix] De Castro, Antonio, et al. "Lactic acid fermentation and storage of blanched garlic." *International Journal of Food Microbiology* Feb. 1998: ScienceDirect Web. Feb. 2015.
[cccx] Sacks, Katherin. "Why does garlic turn blue?" *Epicurious* July 2015: epicurious Web. Sept. 2015.
[cccxi] Cho, Jungeun, et al. "Indentification of candidate amino acids involved in the fermentation of blue pigments in crushed garlic cloves." *Journal of Food Science* Nov. 2008: onlinelibrary.wiley Web. Feb. 2015.
[cccxii] Ibid.
[cccxiii] Bai, B, et al. "Mechanism of the greening color formation of 'laba' garlic, a traditional homemade chinese food product." *Journal of Agricultual and Food Chemistry* Sept. 2005: NCBI Web. Jan. 2015.
[cccxiv] Moore, Michelle. "Garlic- an ancient remedy with a modern twist." *Staph Infection Resources*: staph-infectionresources Web. Nov. 2015.
[cccxv] Cutler, R.R. and P. Wilson. "Antibacterial activity of a new, stabel, aqueous extract of allicin against methicillinresistant Staphylococcus aureus." *British Journal of Biomedical Science* Feb. 2004: NCBI Web. Nov. 2015.
[cccxvi] Fallon, Sally. 2011: (September 2). The Oiling of America. Retrieved from https://www.youtube.com/watch? v=fvKdYUCUca8 (1:23:45).
[cccxvii] Bacic, Melissa and C. Jeffrey Smith. "Laboratory Maintenance and Cultivation of Bacteroides Species." *Current Protocols in Microbiology* May 2008: onlinelibrary.wiley Web. Oct. 2015.
[cccxviii] Gill, Navkiran, et al. "Roadblocks in the gut: barriers in interric infection." *Cellular Microbiology* Mar. 2011: onlinelibrary.wiley Web. Jan. 2011.
[cccxix] Caplan, M.S. and T. Jilling. "Neonatal necrotizing enterocolitis: possible role of probiotic supplementation." *Journal of Pediatric Gastroenterology and Nutrition* 2000: NCBI Web. Jan. 2015.

[cccxx] "Bifidobacteria." *Medline Plus*: medlineplus.gov Web. Jan. 2015.
[cccxxi] Marreau, Philippe R. et al. "Protection from gastrointestinal diseases with the use of probiotics." *The American Journal of Clinical Nutrition* Feb. 2001: ajcn.nutrition Web. Jan. 2015.
[cccxxii] Reid, Gregor. "The Scientific Basis for Probiotic Strains of Lactobacillus." *Applied and Environmental Microbiology* Sept. 1999: NCBI Web. Jan. 2015.
[cccxxiii] Marreau, Philippe R. et al. "Protection from gastrointestinal diseases with the use of probiotics." *The American Journal of Clinical Nutrition* Feb. 2001: ajcn.nutrition Web. Jan. 2015.
[cccxxiv] Thang, Cin L., et al. "Effect of Lactobacillus rhamnosus GG supplementation on cow's milk allergy in mouse model." *Asthma, Allergy & Clinical Nutrition* Dec. 2011: aacijournal.biomedcentral Web. Jan. 2015.
[cccxxv] Tang, Mimi L.K., et al. "Administration of a probiotic with peanut oral immunotherapy: A randomized trial." *The Journal of Allergy and Clinical Nutrition* Mar. 2015: jacionline Web. Oct. 2015.
[cccxxvi] Tomioka, H., et al. "The protective activity of immunostimulants against Listeria monocytogenes infection in mice." *Microbiology Society* Feb. 1992: microbiologyresearch.org Web. Jan. 2015.
[cccxxvii] Mareau, Philippe R., et al. "Protection from gastorintestinal diseases with the use of probiotics." *The American Journal of Clinical Nutrition* Feb. 2001: acjn.nutrition Web. Jan. 2015.
[cccxxviii] Kelesidis, Theodoros and Charalabos Pothoulakis. "Efficacy and safety of the probiotic Saccharomyces boulardii for the prevention and therapy of gastrointestinal disorders." *Therapeutic Advances in Gastroenterology* Mar. 2012: NCBI Web. Jan. 2015.
[cccxxix] Deans, Emily. "Groovy Probiotics." *Psychology Today* June 2012: psychologytoday Web. Feb. 2015.
[cccxxx] Messaoudi, Michael, et al. "Assessment of psychotropic-like properties of a probiotic formulation (Lactobacillus helveticus R0052 and Bificobacterium longum RO175) in rats and human subjects." *British Journal of Nutrition* Mar. 2011: cambridge.org Web. Jan. 2015.
[cccxxxi] Ruiz-Barba, J.L., et al. "Use of Lactobacillus plantrum LPCO10, a Bacteriocin Producer, as a Starter Culture in SpanishStyle Green Olive Fermentations." *Applied and Environmental Microbiology* June 1994: aem.asm Web. Jan. 2015. 332
[cccxxxii] McBride, Natasha. "Gut and Psychology Syndrome (GAPS)." Wise Traditions Conference. London, England. 2012.
[cccxxxiii] Ibid.
[cccxxxiv] "Prescript-Assist Broad Spectrum Probiotic." Prescript Asssist: prescript-assist Web. June 2015.
[cccxxxv] "Biokult": bio-kult Web. June 2015. 336 - "Living Streams Probiotic." Living Streams Mission: Living Streams Web. June 2015.
[cccxxxvi] Ibid.

[cccxxxvii] Cummings, J.H. and G.T. Macfarlane. "Gastrointestinal effects of probiotics." *The British Journal of Nutrition* May 2002: NCBI Web. June 2015.
[cccxxxviii] McBride, Natasha. *Gut and Psychology Syndrome, Natural Treatment for Autism, Dyspraxia, A.D.D., Dyslexia, A.D.H.D., Depression, Schizophrenia.* Cambridge: Medinform Publishing, 2012. Print.
[cccxxxix] McBride, Natasha. "Gut and Psychology Syndrome." Annual Wise Traditions Conference. Anaheim, California. 2015. Lecture.
[cccxl] Ibid.
[cccxli] Ibid.
[cccxlii] Ibid.
[cccxliii] "The Best Probiotic Supplement: It's a jungle in there." *Reviews.com* Dec. 2016: reviews.com Web. Dec. 2016.
[cccxliv] Burdock, George A., et al. "The importance of GRAS to the functional food and nutraceutical industries." Toxicology Apr. 2006: sciencedirect Web. Dec. 2016.
[cccxlv] Neltner, T.G., et al. "Conflicts of interest in approvals of additives to food determined to be generally recognized as safe: out of balance." *JAMA Internal Medicine* Dec. 2013: NCBI Web. Dec. 2015.
[cccxlvi] Wendee, Nicole. "Secret Ingredients: Who Knows What's in Your Food?" *Environmental Health Perspectives* April 2013: ehp.niehs.nih Web. Feb. 2013.
[cccxlvii] Shames, Lisa. "FDA should strengthen its oversight of food ingredients determeind to be Generally Recognizes as Safe (GRAS)." U.S. Government Accountability Office March 2010: gao.gov Web. Feb. 2015.
[cccxlviii] "FDA Investigation Finds 'Unlisted' Ingredients in Food." *California Healthling Daily Edition*: californiahealthline.org Web. Nov. 2016.
[cccxlix] "Opinion of the Scientific Panel on Food Additives, Flavourings, Processing Aids and Materials in Contract with Food (AFC) on a request from the Commission related to Ethyl Cellulose as a food additive." *The EFSA Journal* Feb. 2004: efsa.europa.eu Web. Jan. 2015.
[cccl] Ibid.
[cccli] Ibid.
[ccclii] Villota, R. and J.G. Hawkes. "Food applications and the toxicological and nutritional implications of amorphous silicon dioxide." *Critical Reviews in Food Science and Nutrition* 1986: NCBI Web. Feb. 2015.
[cccliii] Ibid.
[cccliv] Ibid.
[ccclv] "Questions & Answers: Big facts on small particles." Akzo Nobel: akzonobel Web. Feb. 2015.
[ccclvi] "What is silica and what can it do for you?" Akzo Nobel: akzonobel Web. Feb. 2015.
[ccclvii] "Azko Nobel: We Create Everyday Essentials." Akzo Nobel: akzonobel Web. 2015.
[ccclviii] Villota, R. and J.G. Hawkes. "Food applications and the toxicological and

nutritional implications of amorphous silicon dioxide." *Critical Reviews in Food Science and Nutrition* 1986: NCBI Web. Feb. 2015.
[ccclix] Yoshida, S.H., et al. "Silicone breast implants: immunotoxic and epidemiologic issues." *Life Sciences* Mar. 1995: NCBI Web. Feb. 2015.
[ccclx] Ibid.
[ccclxi] "Crystalline silica and health from a European health perspective." Crystalline Silica: crystallinesilica.eu Web. Nov. 2015. http://www.crystallinesilica.eu/content/what-respirable-crystalline-silica-rcs
[ccclxii] Ibid.
[ccclxiii] Ibid.
[ccclxiv] "What is silica?" The European Association of Industrial Silica Producers: eurosil.eu Web. Nov. 2015.
[ccclxv] Loomis, Howard F. *Enzymes, The Key to Health.* Madison, WI: 21st Century Publishing, 2005. Print. pXXVI
[ccclxvi] Ibid. p. 60.
[ccclxvii] Chauhan, Yuvraj P., et al. "Microcrystalline cellulose from cotton rages (waste from garment and hosiery industries)." *International Journal of Chemical Sciences* Feb. 2009: sadgurupublications Web. Jan. 2015.
[ccclxviii] Ibid.
[ccclxix] Rojas, John, et al. "Evaluation of several microcrystalline celluloses obtained from agricultural by-products." *Journal of Advanced Pharmaceutical Technology and Research* July-Sept. 2011: NCBI Web. Jan. 2015.
[ccclxx] Ohwoavworhua, F.O. and T. A. Adelakun. "Non-wood Fibre Production of Microcrystalline Cellulose from Sorghum caudatum: Characterisation and Tableting Properties." *Indian Journal of Pharmaceutical Sciences* May-Jun. 2010: NCBI Web. Feb. 2015.
[ccclxxi] "Microcrystalline Cellulose." *Drugs.com*: drugs.com Web. Jan. 2015.
[ccclxxii] Setu, Nurul Islam, et al. "Preparation of Micrcrystalline Cellulose from Cotton and its Evaluation as Direct Compressible Excipient in the Formulation of Naproxen Tablets." *Bangladesh Journals Online* Dec. 2014: Banglajol.info Web. Jan. 2015.
[ccclxxiii] Ibid.
[ccclxxiv] Ibid.
[ccclxxv] "Final Decision Document: TSCA Section 5(H)(4) Exemption for Acetobacter aceti." EPA 1994: epa.gov Web. Feb. 2015.
[ccclxxvi] Olempska-Beer, Zofia. "Alpha-amylase from Bacillus licheniformis containing a genetically engineered alphaamylase gene from B. licheniformis (thermostable) Chemical and Technical Assessment." Joint FAO/WHO Expert Committee on Food Additives (JECFA)." 2004: foa.org Web. Feb. 2015.
[ccclxxvii] "Final Decision Document: TSCA Section 5(H)(4) Exemption for Acetobacter aceti." EPA 1994: epa.gov Web. Feb. 2015.
[ccclxxviii] Oggioni, Marco Rinaldo, et al. "Recurrent Septicemia in an Immunocompromised Patient Due to Probiotic Strains of Bacillus subtilis."

Journal of Clinical Microbiology Jan. 1998: jcm.asm Web. Jan. 2015.
[ccclxxix] Ibid.
[ccclxxx] Ibid.
[ccclxxxi] Moazzam, Alan A. "Chronic lymphocytic leukemia with central nervous system involvement: Report of two cases with a comprehensive literature review." *Journal of Neuro-Oncology July* 2011: researchgate Web. Jan. 2015.
[ccclxxxii] McBride, Natasha. *Gut and Psychology Syndrome, Natural Treatment for Autism, Dyspraxia, A.D.D., Dyslexia, A.D.H.D., Depression, Schizophrenia*. Cambridge: Medinform Publishing, 2012. Print.
[ccclxxxiii] Brisson, John. "HSO's Part6 – What About Enterococcus faecalis?" *Fix Your Gut*: fixyourgut Web. Nov. 2016.
[ccclxxxiv] Ibid.
[ccclxxxv] Kresser, Chris. "RHR: Treating SIBO, Cold Thermogenesis, and When to Take Probiotics." *Chris Kresser* Mar. 2013: chriskresser Web. Jan. 2014.
[ccclxxxvi] Katz, Sandor. *Wild Fermentation*. White River Junction, Vermont: Chelsea Green Publishing Company, 2003. Print.
[ccclxxxvii] Myers, Amy. "Everything you need to know about histamine intolerance." *mbg Mind Body Green* Oct. 2013: mindbodygreen Web. Jan. 2015.
[ccclxxxviii] Myers, Amy. *The Autoimmune Solution: Prevent and Reverse the Full Spectrum of Inflammatory Symptoms and Diseases.* San Francisco: HaperOne, 2015. Print.
[ccclxxxix] Ibid.
[cccxc] "The Dehydration Allergy Connection." *Water Cures*: watercures.org Web. Sept. 2016.
[cccxci] Ibid.
[cccxcii] "L-histidine." *Amino Acids Studies*: aminoacidsstudies.org Web. Nov. 2016.
[cccxciii] Russell, Robert, et al. "Histidine." *Amino Acid Properties* 2003: russellab Web. Sept. 2016.
[cccxciv] McBride, Natasha. "GAPS Practitioner Training." Orlando Certified GAPS Practitioner Training Course. Orlando. October 2015. Participatory Lecture.
[cccxcv] "L-histidine." *Amino Acids Studies*: aminoacidsstudies.org Web. Nov. 2016.
[cccxcvi] Maintz, Laura and Natalija Novak. "Histamine and histamine intolerance." *The American Journal of Clinical Nutrition* May 2007: ajcnnutrition Web. Jan. 2014.
[cccxcvii] Naidoo, P. and J. Pellow. "A randomized placebo-controlled pilot study of Cat saliva 9cH and Histaminum 9cH in cat allergic adults." *Homeopathy: The Journal of the Faculty of Homeopathy* Apr. 2013: NCBI Web. Feb. 2014.
[cccxcviii] Ibid.
[cccxcix] Tsafrir, Judy. "GAPS, FODMAPS and Histamine Intolerance." Judy Tsafrir: Holistic Adult and Child Psychology in Newton, MA Sept. 2012: Web. Judytsafrirmd Jan. 2014.
[cd] Campbell-McBride, Natasha. "Frequently Asked Questions." Gut and Pshychology Syndrome: gaps.me Web. Dec. 2015.
[cdi] Ibid.
[cdii] Ibid.

[cdiii] Ibid.
[cdiv] Ibid.
[cdv] Ibid.
[cdvi] Ibid.
[cdvii] Allen, Patricia. "Gut and Psychology Snydrome: GAPS." Chattnooga, Weston A. Price Fall Training. Chattanooga. October 2011. Participatory Lecture.
[cdviii] Ibid.
[cdix] Deans, Emily. "Groovy Probiotics." *Psychology Today* June 2012: psychologytoday Web. Feb. 2015.
[cdx] Shistar, Terry. "Antibiotics in Fruit Production A challenge to organic integrity." *Beyond Pesticides* Summer 2011: beyondpesticides.org Web. Aug. 2015.
[cdxi] Godoy, Maria. "A battle over antibiotics in organic apple and pear farming." *NPR* April 2013: npr.org Web. Feb. 2014.
[cdxii] Cimitile, Matthew. "Worried about antibiotics in your beef? Vegetables may not be no better." *Scientific American* Jan. 2009: scientificamerican Web. Feb. 2014.
[cdxiii] "Allergic reaction to antibiotic residues in foods? You may have to watch what your fruits and veggies eat." *Science Dailey* Sept. 2014: sciencedaily Web. Oct. 2014.
[cdxiv] Doheny, Kathleen. "Drugs in our drinking water? Experts put potential risks in perspective after a report that drugs are in the water supply." WebMB: webmd.com Web. Oct. 2014.
[cdxv] Kate and Justin extremehealthradio. 2015: (May 30). Dr. Natasha Campbell-McBride Gut Health Digestion. Retrieved from https://www.youtube.com/watch?v=BsHzydqWoKU (36:12).
[cdxvi] Ibid. (35:50).
[cdxvii] Ibid. (37:24).
[cdxviii] Ibid. (37:50).
[cdxix] Hill, Ray. Propolis, The Natural Antibiotic. UK: Harper Collins Distribution Services. 1977. Print.
[cdxx] Green, James. *The Male Herbal: The Definitive Health Care Book for Men and Boys.* Berkely, California: Crossing Press. 2007. Print.
[cdxxi] Ibid.
[cdxxii] "Colloidal Silver." WebMD: webmd Web. Sept. 2016.
[cdxxiii] Ibid.
[cdxxiv] "Garlic." *Therapy*: therapy.epnet.com Web. Sept. 2016.
[cdxxv] Mandal, Manisha Deb and Mandal Shyamapada. "Honey: it's medicinal property and antibacterial acitvity." *Asian Pacific Journal of Tropical Biomedicine April* 2011: NCBI Web. Feb. 2015.
[cdxxvi] Ibid.
[cdxxvii] McBride, Natasha. *Gut and Psychology Syndrome, Natural Treatment for Autism, Dyspraxia, A.D.D., Dyslexia, A.D.H.D., Depression, Schizophrenia.* Cambridge: Medinform Publishing, 2012. Print. Page 251.

[cdxxviii] Ibid. Page 251.
[cdxxix] Ibid. Pages 50-51.
[cdxxx] "Ethanol." PubChem An Open Chemistry Database: pubchem.ncbi.nlm.nih.gov Web. June 2016.
[cdxxxi] Ibid.
[cdxxxii] McBride, Natasha. *Gut and Psychology Syndrome, Natural Treatment for Autism, Dyspraxia, A.D.D., Dyslexia, A.D.H.D., Depression, Schizophrenia.* Cambridge: Medinform Publishing, 2012. Print. Page 51.
[cdxxxiii] Ibid.
[cdxxxiv] Carey, Emily, et al. "Nonalcoholic Fatty Liver Disease." *Cleveland Clinic, Center for Continuing* Education March 3013: clevelandclinicmeded Web. Jan. 2016.
[cdxxxv] Peterson, Jeffrey D., et al. "Glutathione levels in antigen-presenting cells modulate Th1 versus Th2 response patterns." *Proceedings of the National Academy of Sciences of the United states of America* Mar. 1998: NCBI Web. Jan. 2014.
[cdxxxvi] Ibid.
[cdxxxvii] Bull-Otterson, Lara, et al. "Metagenomic analyses of Alcohol Induced Pathogenic Alterations in the Intetinal Microbiome and the Effect of Lactobacillus rhamnosus GG Treatment." *PLOS One* Jan. 2013: journals.plos.org Web. Jan. 2014.
[cdxxxviii] Ibid.
[cdxxxix] McBride, Natasha. "Gut and Psychology Syndrome." Annual Wise Traditions Conference. Anaheim, California. 2015. Lecture.
[cdxl] Kate and Justin extremehealthradio. 2015: (May 30). Dr. Natasha Campbell-McBride Gut Health Digestion. Retrieved from https://www.youtube.com/watch?v=BsHzydqWoKU (15:25).
[cdxli] Ibid.
[cdxlii] Wedro, Benjamin. "Stool Color, Changes in Color, Texture, and Form." *MedicineNet.com*: medicinenet.net Web. Sept. 2016.
[cdxliii] "Blood in stool." WebMD: webmd Web. June 2016.
[cdxliv] Picco, Michael F. "Stool color: When to worry. Yesterday my stool color turned bright green. Should I be concerned?" *Mayo Clinic*: mayoclinic.org Web. June 2016.
[cdxlv] Ibid.
[cdxlvi] Samach, Michael. "Answers." *Health Tap*: healthtap Web. June. 2016.
[cdxlvii] Jobst, D. and K. Kraft. "Candida species in stool, symtoms and complaints in general practice – a cross-section study of 308 outpatients." *Mycoses* Sept. 2006: NCBI Web. June 2015.
[cdxlviii] Campbell-McBride, Natasha. 2011: (April 2). *GAPS Diet Journey*. Retrieved from http://www.immunitrition.com/GAPS_Practitioner_Traini.html playlist 2/6 5:30
[cdxlix] Goodman, Sara. "Tests Find More Than 200 Chemicals in Newborn Umbilical Cord Blood. Study commissioned by environmental group finds high levels of chemicals in U.S. minority infants." *Scientific American* Dec. 2009:

---

scinetificamerican Web. May 2015.
[cdl] Reinberg, Steven. "Colic: Study." WebMD Jan. 2014: webmd Web. Dec. 2015.
[cdli] Gates, Donna. *Body Ecology Diet.* California: Hay House Publishing, 2010. Print.
[cdlii] Ibid.
[cdliii] Heitz, David. "Probiotic May Prevent Acid Reflux, Constipation, and Colic in Infants." *Healthline News* Jan. 2014: healthlinenews Web. Feb. 2015.
[cdliv] Sung, Valerie. "Probiotics to Prevent or Treat Excessive Infant Crying Systemic Review and Meta-analysis." *The JAMA Network* Dec. 2013: jamanetwork Web. June 2015.
[cdlv] Campbell-McBride, Natasha. 2011: (April 2). *GAPS Diet Journey*. Retrieved from http://www.immunitrition.com/GAPS_Practitioner_Traini.html playlist 2/6 5:45
[cdlvi] Bjamsholt, Thomas. "Bacteria and Chronic Infections." University of Copenhagen, Coursera. Web. 2005. Lecture.
[cdlvii] Ibid.
[cdlviii] Ibid.
[cdlix] Ibid.
[cdlx] Ibid.
[cdlxi] Ibid.
[cdlxii] Cook, Ken. 2012: (July 23). 10 Americans. Retrieved from http://www.ewg.org/news/videos/10-americans
[cdlxiii] Goodman, Sarah. "Tests Find More Than 200 Chemicals in Newborn Umbilibal Cord Blood." *Scientific American* Dec. 2009: scientificamerican Web. Jan. 2014.
[cdlxiv] "Polychlorinated biphenyls (PCBs)." *Breast Cancer Fund:* breastcancerfund Web. Jan. 2016.
[cdlxv] White, Heather. The Autoimmune Summit. Web. 2016. Lecture.
[cdlxvi] Ibid.
[cdlxvii] "Safe Drinking Water Act." *EPA*: epa.gov Web. July 2016.
[cdlxviii] White, Heather. The Autoimmune Summit. Web. 2016. Lecture.
[cdlxix] Ibid.
[cdlxx] Hawthorne, Michael. "Testing shows treated foam offers no safety benefit. Fire-resistant barriers may do a better job, cut chemical exposure." *Chicago Tribune* May 2012: articles.chicagotribune Web. Apr. 2012.
[cdlxxi] "Limiting Lead in Lipstick and Other Cosmetics." *U.S. Food and Drug Administration*: fda.gov Web. May 2016.
[cdlxxii] Kiernan, Bill, Global Ag Invention: globalaginvention Web. Aug. 2015.
[cdlxxiii] Ibid.
[cdlxxiv] *Merck Veterinarian Manual.* Georgia: Merck & Co., 2012. Print.
[cdlxxv] Sarich, Christine. "First long-term study released on pigs, cattle who eat GMO soy and corn offers frightening results." *Nation of Change* Jul. 2013: sott.net

Web. Feb. 2014.

[cdlxxvi] Ibid.

[cdlxxvii] Ibid.

[cdlxxviii] Ibid.

[cdlxxix] Ibid.

[cdlxxx] Yong, Ed. "Power lines disrupt the magnetic alignment of cows and deer." *Science Blogs* Mar. 2009: scienceblog.com Web. Aug. 2014.

[cdlxxxi] Angell, R.F., et al. "Effects of a High-Voltage Direct-Current Transmission Line on Beef Cattle Production." *Bioelectromagnetics* 1990: oreganstate.edu Web. Mar. 2012.

[cdlxxxii] Hillman, Donald, et al. "Electric and Magnetic Fields (EMF) Affect Production and Behavior of Cows; Results Using Shielded Neutral Isolation Transformer." *Shocking News* July 2004: electricalpollution Web. Feb. 2013.

[cdlxxxiii] W. Löscher and G. Käs. "Conspicuous behavioral abnormalities in a dairy cow herd near a TV and Radio transmitting antenna." *Practical Veterinary Surgeon* 1998: whale.to/b/loscher.html Web. Jul. 2012.

[cdlxxxiv] Ibid.

[cdlxxxv] Herbert, Martha. Healthy Gut Summit. Web. 2016. Lecture.

###